The Writer's Workbook

The Writer's Workbook
Health Professionals Guide to Getting Published

Shirley H. Fondiller, EdD, RN

National League for Nursing Press • New York
Pub. No. 14-2470

This book was set in Palatino by Publications Development Company of Texas.

The editor and designer was Allan Graubard.

Northeastern Press was the printer and binder.

Cover design by Lillian Welsch.

Printed in the United States of America.

To my son, David,
for continuing so ably
the family tradition of journalism

Contents

Preface   *ix*
Acknowledgments   *xi*
Foreword   *xiii*

PART 1

Introduction   3
Lessons
  1. The Right Idea and What Comes Next   5
  2. Collecting Your Data   17
  3. How to Develop Your Article   27
  4. The Dynamic Duo: Organizing and Outlining   39
  5. The Query Letter—What's It All About?   49
  6. The "Catchy" Lead to Logical Conclusion   61
  7. The Moment of Truth: Your First Draft   73
  8. How to Be Your Own Editor   83
  9. Behind the Editor's Desk   91
  10. Ethics in Journalism: What Health Professionals Need to Know   105

Selected Bibliography on Professional Writing   119

Answers to Self-Test Questions   121

PART 2

Your Assignments: What You Need to Know   131

PART 3

Do's and Don'ts of Modern Usage   169
Common Proofreader's Marks   173
List of Nursing Journals   175

Preface

*T*he Writer's Workbook is just what you have been waiting for! No need to resist any longer that desire to publish. Here is the perfect guide to take you from the very beginning stages into the successful world of health care journalism.

Although the workbook offers some helpful hints on modern usage and style, it is not a primer on grammar and composition. It deals with the writing process through a series of practical lessons enhanced by self-tests and assignments. Although the text contains examples that may appear more relevant to nurses, it can be extremely useful to other health professionals eager to publish.

Designed primarily for the novice writer in the health field, the workbook also gives some timely tips to the more seasoned author on "struggling" less and producing more and better. Informally written in a logical, orderly fashion, it shows the reader how the principles used in preparing articles for publication are the same principles to be followed in most kinds of professional writing, from term papers to theses.

You know better than anyone the importance of communicating well in writing, whether it is the documentation on a patient's chart or a memo to a colleague. Cultivating the craft of writing in its many forms, particularly in the publishing arena, will be a big plus in advancing your career.

Shirley H. Fondiller, EdD, RN

Acknowledgments

With this *Writer's Workbook,* I happily surrender to the wishes of my students and others. For years I ignored their pleas for a better book. Besides, as a teacher of writing, my students had the benefit of feedback to their progress in my courses and writing clinics.

I am grateful to all my students, from whom I learned firsthand about the needs and concerns of health professionals eager to publish. Some will see their own situations reflected in the pages of this workbook. I revel in the scholarship of many of these young authors who will continue to publish.

A special thank you is extended to Dr. Suzanne S. Blancett, a fine editor and writer in the nursing field, who reviewed part of the manuscript and gave invaluable insights. Also, I express my appreciation to Thomas G. Goss, former managing editor of the *American Journal of Nursing,* for his wise counsel, particularly on the editorial process.

I am deeply indebted to Barbara Jo Nerone, colleague and friend, who critiqued the entire manuscript and offered some telling observations.

Finally, I wish to acknowledge Sally Barhydt, managing editor and assistant vice president, National League for Nursing Press, whose professionalism and patience guided the work along this exciting journey into journalism.

Foreword

*I*nside every nurse is the desire to be a published author. For most nurses, however, the wish to contribute to nursing and receive recognition for accomplishments through publishing remains a dream.

Unlike those nurses who don't get published, often because they never try or because they cannot deal creatively with a manuscript rejection, you are on the road to becoming a published author. The fact that you have started reading this workbook is the first step in the process of writing for publication.

Over the years, I have spoken to thousands of nurses about publishing. What frequently deters them from writing is lack of knowledge about how to get started and fear of the unknown. Those who try and don't succeed most often have their manuscripts rejected because content was unfocused, already well discussed in the literature, not relevant to the appropriate readership, or poorly developed and written.

This workbook will help you avoid these common reasons for not getting published. The book's step-by-step approach makes it easy to begin. It demystifies the writing and publishing process, which is simpler than it may seem. If time is taken to break the process down into its elemental steps, apparent difficulties can become building blocks.

Too often books intended to help nurses write for publication are written at a complex and academic level; they often present too much information, overwhelming would-be-authors with nice-to-know rather than need-to-know advice. The book I always recommended to nurse authors is now out of print, but I'm happy to say this workbook is a better guide for nurses and will be my new recommendation.

The ability to practice what you learn is critical to success in any task. Unlike other books on writing for publication, this book gives the reader assignments to complete following each chapter. Whether you use the assignments as a self-learning tool or take advantage of the author's program to critique your work, you will learn to approach the writing process in a logical, straightforward manner and you will be motivated to continue. Since the steps every author takes when writing remain the same, you will continue to use what you learn even as you become more confident and accomplished.

Writing for publication is a process that can be learned and can be mastered. Enjoy this workbook, savor its lessons, welcome the experience of learning something new. And finally, relish the thrill of seeing your name in print and helping advance nursing knowledge through your publications. I look forward to reading your article!

Suzanne Smith Blancett, EdD, RN
Editor-in-Chief
Journal of Nursing Administration
and *Nurse Educator*
J. B. Lippincott Company
Philadelphia, Pennsylvania

Part 1

Introduction

HOW TO USE THIS BOOK

*P*eople who want to become writers don't get there by wish, hope, or even dreams. They *earn* their glory. As part of every successful author's armamentarium, these basic qualities dominate: *curiosity, good manners, style, and perseverance.* Follow the example of Eugene O'Neill when he said: "I am a dramatist . . . . What I see everywhere in life is drama." Who better than nurses and other health professionals can speak to and write about the drama that occurs almost every day in the worlds of practice, education, management, and research. So, be curious, ask questions, and keep a log if you want to write. Record the dialogue of patients and others as it will add vitality to that article you are yearning to write.

For simplicity of style, turn to the eloquent prose of Katherine Anne Porter, who explained that the mission of a writer was to purify the language. "Don't use words you have look up in the dictionary," she once cautioned students during one of her lectures. For terse, crisp writing, spend some time reading Hemingway's short stories. He was a master of stripping words to their bare bones.

Finally, perhaps the most important quality of a writer is that of perseverance. If you tend to procrastinate, other rewards may come your way but authorship will not be one of them. Writing, and then rewriting—an even more essential skill—requires self-discipline and an agonizing "stick-to-itiveness."

Keep in mind that in many journals you will be writing primarily for the practicing professional rather than the theoretician. Therefore, you need to supplement your article with anecdotes, real-life experience, dialogue, and quotations or references.

Your readers are not seeking a procedural manual but practical information, the "how-to's," on health delivery patterns, clinical interventions, management information systems, creative approaches to staffing, computer innovations, teaching strategies, and so on.

Although there is always a place for new interpretations and opinion pieces, writing on controversial topics can be risky for beginners. Leave those articles to the "pros"—knowledgeable and established authors who can handle them.

Through illustration, *show* (not tell) your audience the who, what, when, where, why, and how of the activity or program you are describing. Share with them the evolution of your idea and its effectiveness, the players involved, the activity's positive features and limitations, and your suggestions for continuing implementation.

Well-written articles offering fresh information, whether slated for practice, education, management, or research journals, give birth to a host of benefits—none the least being the satisfaction derived from seeing your work in print. More significantly, however, is the response from readers impressed with your article, who may seek to replicate or adapt your project or study to their own settings. The published work, whether an article or book, thus becomes a powerful force in advancing a profession. It is from such sources in the health care field that newer movements have evolved. In nursing, for example, just look at the published work on case management in nursing practice, computer assisted instruction, interactive video in education, and the growing trend of nurse entrepreneurship sweeping communities nationwide.

The lessons in this *Writer's Workbook* will help you earn your claim to authorship. Study each lesson carefully, and take each self-test to determine your understanding of what you have just read. What follows is the most exciting aspect of this unique program: *an assignment with each lesson that will carry you into the next phase of the writing process by providing individual feedback (if you choose the option) from an editorial expert in the health care field.*

In a sense, you will be studying in a classroom without walls, able to write at your own pace and on your own turf. You will be guided by a recognized writer and editor associated with *Publishing for Health Dimensions-phd*, an editorial service for nurses and health professionals. *Phd*, which advises and assists with placement, will be happy to work with you throughout the program, or in selected lessons as needed, through correspondence and other forms of communication.

Remember *writing is work*. But when you follow the process in an orderly, progressive way, the lessons will come naturally. By the time you're completing one article, you will already be thinking about that next article.

We wish you luck in publishing and hope that you will let *The Writer's Workbook* and *phd* guide you through another challenging adventure in your career.

Lesson 1

The Right Idea and What Comes Next

"How do I get started? I think I have a good idea for an article but I don't know where to begin!"

Sound familiar? Of course. But perk up, you have lots of company—neophyte writers as well as many of your more seasoned contemporaries. Once you learn the process, however, you will triumph over that seemingly insurmountable obstacle and quietly gloat, having penetrated the so-called mystique of a beginning writer's block. After all, bigger barriers have been conquered before. Just think about landing on the moon!

Keep in mind that unless you're a literary wiz or a miracle worker, you just can't sit down at your computer or typewriter, or however you write, and expect to dash off the long overdue opus you've been dreaming about. You will need form and a format, in short, a systematic approach to your article.

Before you begin to ruminate about an appropriate topic, never lose sight of this important adage: *Write what you know about.* Yours is a rich background in your field, so share those experiences with colleagues. Sure, you may have a yen to write a gothic or romantic novel ("I can write as well as Danielle Steel"—well, maybe), but first earn some credibility in your own profession before expanding to other markets.

When planning an article, you will want to share something with your readers that is worth sharing. From the outset, you should have some notion of your destination. After all, an artist doesn't start a picture by dabbing paint on a canvas, hoping that a portrait will emerge out of colored blobs. Nor does an architect begin a building before working out the details on a drawing board.

Perhaps your concept is already clear in your mind since you have been thinking about it for some time. More likely, however, it may still be a bit fuzzy, requiring a gestation period to grow clearer. Remember, all you need for one good article is *one* good topic. Don't get bogged down with two or more topics. Tuck them away in your "Future Articles" file.

Prior to firming up your topic, be sure to explore the professional literature within the previous two years (a reasonable period) to discover any articles similar to the article you are proposing. You will, of course, be disappointed if you find that the journal of your choice has featured a piece in this general area three months earlier. Although your slant may differ somewhat, your best bet would be to consider another publication. Fortunately, the health care market is extensive, with some journals competing for the same types of articles.

In addition to culling out "repeats," a search will provide you with background information or documentation that may be useful in developing your idea. But hold off on the notetaking until you have a good handle on your central focus.

To help firm up your topic, study carefully the questions below. How they are addressed determines whether a prospective author has selected a viable concept and is on the right track to a potentially marketable article. As the first step in the writing process, focusing on an appropriate topic is crucial because it provides the foundation for all other steps to follow.

WHAT IS THE CENTRAL THRUST OF MY ARTICLE?

In other words, what message do you wish to express to your audience? By thinking your idea through clearly, you should be able to express it clearly. If that is easier said than done, then here is something to help you.

Why not start with a thesis statement? Broadly speaking, a thesis statement informs the reader of your main idea (Gehle & Rollo, 1987). A thesis also shows the care you have given to planning the article. It will evolve from your topic and by addressing the following questions: (1) *What* is my point? (2) *How* will I present it? (3) *Why* is my point important? Study the example below.

THE RIGHT IDEA AND WHAT COMES NEXT

TOPIC

Why nurses in a privately-funded nurse-managed teen center, affiliated with a midwestern university hospital, are key people to provide high-risk adolescents with education and counseling on sexuality and reproductive issues.

WHY IS MY POINT IMPORTANT?

The teen center described can serve as a model for comparable sites and populations in the nation.

HOW WILL I PRESENT IT?

By showing how a nurse-managed teen center in a large mid-western community is helping to educate teenagers on sexuality and reproduction issues through special programs, classes, individual counseling, and referrals.

WHAT IS MY POINT?

To educate a high-risk population in which AIDS and venereal disease are on the increase along with the number of unwed teenage mothers, many of whom deliver infants with crack, potential H.I.V. infection, and other disorders.

THESIS

The rise of life-threatening illnesses, such as AIDS among inner city adolescents has demonstrated their lack of education or understanding in this area as well as other health problems relating to sexuality and reproduction. Through creative programs, counseling, and referral, nurse practitioners and staff in a nurse-managed teen center have developed a model to reach this population with encouraging results to date.

Your thesis may be expressed in one or more sentences depending on the topic's complexity. Although some editors may be interested in a broad-based article such as the one proposed above, other editors may prefer limiting the content to a particular service or program within the teen center. (That is why letters of query and proposals are important. See Lesson 5.) Suggested are two topics with a narrower focus that should allow for adequate substance and exposition:

1. Nurse-managed teen center implements innovative interactive video program on family planning for inner city girls and boys.

2. Nurse-managed center spearheads interdisciplinary AIDs education program with promising results for inner city teens and families.

7

Each of the two topics has marketable potential. The appeal is in their specificity. Both ideas reflect a "how-to" approach, showing the reader the sequential development of a concept through completion. In effect, the author is saying: "We have introduced a program that works. Perhaps you, too, would like to try it."

So, narrowing your idea to a particular procedure, technique, or program can propel you into publishing if the piece is fresh, interesting, and well presented.

Arriving at a workable topic will take some thought. Once you firm up your focus, however, you'll be on your way. Expanding technology, computerization, and significant research have not only generated but demanded new modalities and protocols in health care, changing services, and greater expertise among all health professionals. A moveable feast of exciting ideas is out there, just waiting for you to put practice into print. Do it and share the wealth!

WHAT IS YOUR TARGET AUDIENCE? WHAT JOURNALS WOULD BE APPROPRIATE?

Before you begin your article, consider this question: Who will benefit from reading your manuscript? The purpose of the work will determine your target audience which, in turn, affects the way it is presented.

With the degree of specialization among some health care disciplines, writers have a plethora of markets to go for, and it sometimes can be difficult to decide on the right journal. As an author in search of an audience, you may be faced with a dilemma. You have a topic in mind, a poignant story to share from your experience, or perhaps significant research to report. You are uncertain, however, where to place the article. The following hypothetical example will provide some clarity.

You are a primary nurse, working on a bone marrow transplant unit, and you suggest the following topic:

To show how peer support, enhanced by the nurse's understanding and expertise, helped two adolescent boys with leukemia to cope with bone marrow transplantation.

Where would you publish this kind of an article? In a journal slated for oncology nurses or in a journal with a more general nursing focus? Largely, that decision will depend on whom and where you wish to make the greatest impact. If you select the journal that reaches a broader audience, whose readers may not be too familiar with the topic, you probably will have to introduce explanatory material.

In another situation, you may be a health systems manager in a tertiary medical center, eager to report on a twelve-month study of interdisciplinary case management piloted on four patient care units. The data show impressive cost-saving features of a new delivery system.

What audience should your article address? Hospital administrators, fiscal officers, physicians, nurse administrators, social workers, or others? First, determine what you want to accomplish in the article. If a broad-based readership is your goal, than you might select *Hospital & Health Services Administration,* a publication that attracts various health professionals. If not, the readers of *Topics in Health Care Financing* may be your perfect target group.

When you decide on your audience, examine scrupulously recent issues of journals targeted to that particular group. You may already have a publication in mind. Scan past issues to observe any changes in format and content direction. Changing editors frequently "sweep clean," bringing in new ideas and generating a brand new look.

Another periodical, *Image—Journal of Nursing Scholarship,* intensified an earlier but more modest thrust on nursing research when Donna Diers came on board as editor. Her strong support of this area is reflected in the pages of every issue of the quarterly.

Your initial task, therefore, is to examine the journal in which you may wish to publish. The nature and length of articles, number of single or multiple authors, writing style, use of first-person "I" approach, and development of the work from its "catchy lead" to logical conclusion are all important aspects in your examination. Furthermore, don't overlook the different departments and the types of illustrations either.

A "must" for all prospective authors is the information sheet available from most health care journals. This resource offers guidelines on manuscript preparation and submission, the review process, payment (if given), photos, and reference format. Some journals carry these guidelines in each issue or periodically. Review them *before* beginning your article.

The idea of expanding your vistas to reach out to new audiences and journals is important for professional people. If you are a beginning author working as a clinician, educator, manager, or researcher, start writing for journals in your particular specialty. In time, when you begin to publish, reach out to the more general journals in the field. But keep that proverbial back burner warming, because some day you will want to share your expertise in publications read by other health professionals as well as by people in the public arena.

IS YOUR ARTICLE MARKETABLE?

So you think you have a terrific idea? Perhaps you do. But not so fast. The real question is—can you sell it?

If you follow the rule of assuming nothing and checking everything, then your chances of success are quite good. Study these pointers.

1. Your Proposed Article Has Not Appeared in Print, Particularly in Recent Months

Although it may be a disquieting thought, two people (and sometimes more) can have the same idea. Therefore, if you've been pondering a potential topic for some time, hustle and begin the real work.

First, however, scan the periodical literature to make sure that the article you're proposing hasn't appeared in print, particularly in recent months. Better to find out now than later. If that should be the case, quickly reactivate your creative juices and start developing your next idea.

2. Your Article Provides New Information

There is a whole new body of literature on the contemporary health care scene, showing the response of imaginative health professionals to the changing environment. As a participant, you will want to capture in writing the remarkable innovations in your own setting. Perhaps you have been involved in a novel staff development program on diabetes education, or implementing a new modality in physical therapy for patients with degenerative joint disease. Perhaps it is time to report your study of the well elderly in urban day care centers.

Also, don't believe that just because an article has a recurring idea it may be unacceptable for publication. When approached with a new twist, or from a fresh perspective, an older topic may continue to hold interest. You must be able to discern the above, however, from an overworked topic, even one of more recent vintage.

For example, experimentation in primary nursing accelerated in the middle 1970s and early 1980s, and produced a rash of articles flooding the journal market. After a while, more than one editor would throw up her hands in despair at the onslaught of "repeats." The common retort: "Not another one on *that* topic!"

Here is a related point on other "no-no's" of editors. The term paper may be academia's gift to the student community but, except in rare cases, it is verboten to professional journals. One of the reasons editors reject these manuscripts is that they rarely contain new information. When students investigate their topic, the material has already appeared in the literature.

3. Your Article Contains Significant Information

Although you consider your article important, you must try to project how others will respond to it. Will your readers find the information of interest? Useful? Will they care?

If you feel passionate about what you want to share, believing that it will make a difference and contribute to your profession, communicate that message to the audience. Your ability to express your idea in a clear, straightforward manner that will reflect its significance will impress your readers and enhance the credibility of your article.

4. Your Article Is Relevant

Nobody is interested in yesterday's news. Journal editors crave articles current with developments in your field. Be familiar with what they want (often spelled out in the guidelines for prospective authors) and then work on your idea within that circumscribed area.

Editors are justifiably dismayed when proposed articles with dated or untimely topics reach their desk. Some pieces are so well written that you wonder at all that good effort gone to waste. "Where have these people been?" asks one editor, commenting on a recent manuscript on progressive patient care. "Why that concept is as old as high button shoes!"

The extensive number of health care journals not only reflects the variety of disciplines and health professionals who read them, but also indicates the respective needs of specific audiences from first line managers to quality assurance coordinators. As an aspiring author, you will want to deal with a problem, program, or practice that has a contemporary slant—perhaps new techniques in scoliosis screening, transplant nursing, staff scheduling, AIDs education in the curriculum, or some other activity.

To paraphrase a popular television show: *You be in touch and your readers will be in touch.*

5. Your Article Is Manageable

When you begin writing your article, you will want to continue at a steady pace until it is completed. Don't select a topic too complex or global or your narrative may run away with itself (and you), leaving that long-sought conclusion in limbo.

This problem, however, can be averted from the outset if you properly define your main idea and its scope. What may seem like an exciting article at the time could take months and months of investigation or involve several trips away from home. Unless your intent is to report a study, temper those lofty aspirations and concentrate on a manageable and realistic topic.

Be familiar with the required length of manuscripts, which differs from journal to journal. Some publications that have experienced a decrease in advertising revenue have reduced by necessity the number of pages. In order to avoid cutting down on the quantity of articles, editors are requesting shorter pieces in such cases.

Journals such as *Nursing* give authors a variety of options as to length. Targeted to the staff nurse, *Nursing* features articles as well as several departments that give beginners an excellent chance to break into print with brief, inciteful stories based largely on personal experience.

Another example, the *Journal of Nursing Administration,* which is designed for top-level nurse administrators, suggests manuscript length from seven to eighteen typed pages. Both *Nursing Research* and *Image* stipulate a maximum number of 3,500 words or fourteen pages. To find out length requirements of most health care journals, your best bet is to read the author guidelines.

WHAT ARE YOUR SOURCES OF INFORMATION?

To do justice to your proposed article, know early in the exploratory phase the kinds of resources to use in developing your topic. Suppose you are a nurse manager on a hospital's medical/surgical unit, which recently implemented a new documentation system using the Carolyn Marker Model. You and your staff are eager to share this information with other nurses. If you have kept a systematic log of the process involved in introducing the model, then your article could almost write itself!

Nevertheless, you will want to supplement the experiential part with other background to add more depth to the work. The chances are that you already acquired considerable data (including a computer search) before proceeding with the new documentation system. It doesn't hurt, however, to return to the literature—books and periodicals—to see if any subsequent material has appeared in the interim. If there is any grist for the mill to enrich your topic, use it!

The practice of maintaining a log in general is a great idea for prospective authors. Get into the habit of recording regularly what you see, hear, or feel in particular situations. Whether you are a nurse, nutritionist, or occupational therapist, observe, listen, and jot down notes on happenings that you may wish to include in an article some day. These entries become precious reminders, adding a human and realistic touch.

Ideas come from unexpected sources. The use of comments by authorities in certain types of articles is often essential—they will enhance your credibility. When appropriate, a big plus is capturing "live" the words of these people either in person or in a telephone interview. This approach takes proper preparation and effective communication skills. Practice and you will become perfect at it (see Lesson 2).

Another resource with publishing potential is a speech or paper presented at a national, state, or local conference. You have often seen the annotation at the bottom of an article's first page indicating something like, "This article was reproduced from a talk given at the annual National Teaching Institute of the American Association of Critical Care Nurses in Boston, May 1991."

So, when preparing a paper for oral presentation, keep in mind that it may be adapted for publication. Don't be surprised, however, if some editing or reworking is necessary in the transition from spoken word to written word.

ARE YOU QUALIFIED TO WRITE THIS ARTICLE?

Above all, the question of an author's qualifications is paramount when considering a published work. If you have been involved in a new procedure, teaching program, pattern of care, or significant research, then who better than you to write about it? It is not unusual for an editor to ask, "Do you have the expertise to do this article?"

The answer, of course, lies in the product (manuscript) itself, although your cover letter will brief the editor on your experience as well as academic background. Your topic must illustrate how the activity you are describing has moved far beyond the conceptual stage. No one is interested in what you think may be a super idea but has yet to be implemented. Instead, show the entire evolution of the effort from inception through completion and then you will have a story to tell.

If you plan to share the publishing spotlight with other colleagues, make certain of their valid claim to authorship. The old saying—"Too many cooks spoil the broth"—can be applied to articles with multiple contributors. Ensure your proper visibility so that editors won't wonder: *Will the real author please stand up?*

SUMMARY

Focusing on an idea in a planned, thoughtful way will hasten your entry into the publishing world. It represents the initial and most difficult step in the writing process because it is the foundation on which you must build to reach your goal: a completed, marketable article.

Answer the Self-Test and see how effective your introductory lesson has been. Then you will be ready to begin your first assignment. You have the option of working on your own or with a team of editorial experts in the health field, who will guide you throughout your lessons with prompt and substantive feedback. (See the assignments at the back of this workbook, which can be coordinated with *phd.*)

The choice is yours. But first, *set a target date to begin your article and, more importantly, a target date to finish!*

LESSON 1

SELF-TEST

Circle the appropriate answer below.   **True False**

1. If the journal of your choice recently featured the topic you had in mind, forget about it and select a new idea.   T   F

2. It is best to delay note taking for an article until the focus of your article is more firmed up.   T   F

3. The major factor in determining whether to slate your article for a specialty or general journal depends on reaching the largest audience.   T   F

4. Reviewing journals over the previous six months is ample time to avoid repeating topics.   T   F

5. Writing for the public is what every health professional should do as soon as possible.   T   F

6. It is best to avoid writing about recurring themes because they never say anything new.   T   F

7. Term papers make good articles if they are well written and well organized.   T   F

8. If your article provides new information and is significant, relevant, and manageable, your chances of marketing it are quite good.   T   F

9. You and your staff are ready to begin phase I of an exciting new program. You would like to share with readers the planning and development process up to this time. Is this a good idea?   T   F

10. Papers presented at conferences or meetings rarely need to be edited for publication.   T   F

Lesson 2

Collecting Your Data

Congratulations! You're now over the hump of that first giant step in the writing process. But you can only move forward if you do your lessons and complete your assignments.

The basic material for your article is there, just waiting for you. Like an investigative reporter, it's time to begin a "digging" process, selectively culling essential data to enhance and substantiate your central idea.

The initial task will be to determine your best sources. As a starter, tap your memory to pluck out what you may already know about the topic. If you are considering a case study approach involving an unusual patient experience, or comparing student responses to a novel computerized self-learning module with a more traditional method, you probably have a good idea of what you want to say. But you will still need some time to recollect and recreate for yourself certain scenes and incidents.

Make a conscious effort to remember half-forgotten details—they will give a vitality to your article. Try to recapture that telling exchange with a patient, colleague, or employer. This retrospective exercise is certain to generate interesting material along with some useful tidbits of information. Be sure to record your thoughts promptly!

Although memory has its place in the creative process, it is only your first source for revealing background information. Journals, books, audio/video tapes, and other reference works are indispensable to acquiring greater depth of understanding of your particular topic.

Another valuable resource, when appropriate, are the comments or opinions of authorities in the field. Learn to sift out those relevant excerpts from the published works of experts that will strengthen your article. In some cases, you may wish to interview the individual either in person or on the telephone if it will add to the work. As an author, you will want to become a good interviewer, whether you need the material for a feature story or a more comprehensive profile.

Your Library: What It Can Do for You

It goes without saying that a library is the *sine qua non* of all writers. To derive maximum benefit from a library, however, you must know what it offers and how to use it.

Whether you decide to use a library located in a private or public institution, health science center, or hospital, you should be aware that its holdings are arranged either by the Dewey decimal system or by the Library of Congress system. Some libraries use both. If you learn the basics of each system, you will be able to find material more easily.

Most libraries contain three broad resources: (1) general reference materials, (2) periodical indexes, and (3) a list of the library's holdings. General reference works include encyclopedias, bibliographies, yearbooks, dictionaries, atlases, and similar works. Although they provide information in various subject areas, don't depend on them for the substance of your paper since they represent a collection of writings done by others.

Periodical literature consists of journals, magazines, or newspapers published on a regular basis. There are several periodical indexes, each of which lists articles published in periodicals on a specific subject or professional area. As a health professional, become familiar with these indexes, such as the quarterly *International Nursing Index,* the bimonthly *Cumulative Index to Nursing and Allied Health,* the monthly *Index Medicus,* and the quarterly *Hospital Literature Index.* Other useful guides are the *Education Index, Social Sciences Index, General Science Index,* and *Humanities Index.*

If you're interested in more general material (including updated health-related topics), consult the newspaper indexes published by the *New York Times,* the *Wall Street Journal,* the *Washington Post,* and the *Christian Science Monitor.*

An easy to use bimonthly is the *Readers Guide to Periodical Literature,* which publishes current articles indexed by author and subject.

Libraries contain a list of holdings that includes books and pamphlets as well as video and audiotapes, films, and other nonprint materials. You will find entries arranged alphabetically under the subject(s), title, and author's name (last name first). The list is usually housed in the card catalog but it may also be on microfiche, microfilm, or microcard. Some libraries, particularly in universities, use a computer data system for storing their holdings, which can be accessed through a computer terminal.

Begin your library exploration by orienting yourself to the available resources and services. Cultivate the librarians, whose support and expertise can ease your load (and anxiety) as you proceed with your article.

If you wish to do a computer search on your topic, reference librarians are great resource people. They will guide you in focusing on key words, which will make all the difference in the kinds of citations identified on your computer printout. In addition, they can recommend the appropriate databases as well as the fee for the search.

Ask about available databases, especially those on health science literature, such as MEDLINE. A word of caution, however, on computer searches. Although they have wide access, they take time. If you're eager to begin, you might be better off pursuing another route. Why not spend several concentrated hours in the library, delving into the periodical indexes? You probably will come up with comparable data.

Compiling a Working Bibliography

As you consult the library's indexes and list of holdings, you will be compiling a working bibliography. From the outset, block out a period of time to perform the task adequately. It is better to spend one, two, or even three days consecutively in the library, in concentrated study, than spacing out the intervals over weeks. Otherwise, you will lose time and possibly motivation.

Depending on the nature of your topic, your search can sometimes get out of hand unless you are selective. It may be a painstaking process, but remember one cardinal rule: *Be in control of your data.* That is, in assembling the material, look for the most relevant and comprehensive works. Be practical. No need to list 50 plus books in the same general area! Be discriminating on what appears promising.

Another tip: Put your critical eye to good use. Some book titles can be misleading in that they imply more than what they deliver. What you may think is a goldmine can turn out to be something quite sketchy and superficial. Weed out those sources early.

Finally, be accurate and thorough as you extract information for your list of works cited. Once engrossed in your article, it should not be necessary to return to the library to add new sources or embellish existing sources. That is a wasteful exercise that can be avoided if you've done your job well.

Although various methods can be employed in completing a working bibliography, you may find the following suggestions helpful. To list your references, use 3 × 5 index cards since they are easier to handle than paper, useful for filing or arranging an outline, and tend to hold up better for prolonged use. One card for each citation is recommended because other index cards (4 × 6), matching a specific citation, will be used for the actual notetaking.

The information below will guide you in developing your working bibliography, which must be completed before taking notes. For citations, you may wish to use the format described in the *Publication Manual of the American Psychological Association,* since many journal and book editors prefer APA style on manuscripts.

Your index card should include:

1. Library call number of a book. Also, cite the author(s), year of publication, title, edition (if not the first), volume (if more than one), place of publication, and publisher.

2. For an article, cite the author(s), year of publication, title, periodical, volume number, issue number, total number of pages.

3. For nonprint material such as a computer software program, cite the writer, title, descriptive label, year of publication, and distributor.

4. For nonprint material such as a recording, cite the composer, title, artist(s) performing the work, conductor, date of recording, and manufacturer's catalog number.

If it will enhance your topic, indicate any further information on the index card. For example, does the reference contain illustrations, a bibliography at the end of each chapter (if a book), interesting appendices, or other pertinent details.

The Art of Notetaking

You may think it presumptuous to suggest how to take notes at this stage of your career. But in preparing an article, notetaking assumes a new dimension. Your chances of successful outlining will depend, to a large extent, on how precise, accurate, and comprehensive you have been in gathering your data.

Notetaking must be functional. Prior to beginning the process, think about some workable headings for your paper. Perhaps you may want to make a cursory or scratch outline reflecting your knowledge of the topic. Start by jotting down your ideas quickly, and forming and arranging the headings in logical order.

Shifting to your other index cards (4 × 6), copy some of the same information from the source card in the working bibliography. Include the author(s) full name and a short form of the work's title. If you're a researcher, you may wish to add a subject heading at the top of the card that will identify its basic content. In some cases, be prepared to use more than one card for a particular source. Always indicate the exact page number of material you are extracting.

Your notes should reflect careful reading and understanding of the source. When recording, be sure to distinguish between facts and opinions. If you are reporting research, write down where and when the study was conducted, materials and equipment used, and results obtained.

Your approach to taking notes will involve summarizing, paraphrasing, and direct quoting. A summary is useful when you want to capture as succinctly as possible some important idea or point of view of a particular article or book.

In paraphrasing, you restate in your own words the essence of what you are extracting. This method increases your understanding of the information, which will be incorporated more easily into your article. Learn to cultivate paraphrasing, a skill all too often discounted by beginning writers who resort instead to excessive quoting. This practice shortchanges the readers and will convince an editor that the author has not done a good job.

Quoting, however, which means reproducing the exact words of the original source, can be extremely effective in certain cases. If you believe an authority's remarks will carry more weight than paraphrasing, or when accurate phrasing is considered important, by all means use this method. Another indicator is when the language of the person being quoted is especially colorful, descriptive, or forceful.

Whenever you summarize, paraphrase, or quote material, be a responsible reporter and give credit where it is due. As a published author, you too will expect this same courtesy.

Getting the Most Out of Experts

If you decide that first-hand comments from authorities will enrich your article, then include them. An interview, whether in person or on the telephone, is one of the most common and popular nonfiction forms. But do some hard thinking well in advance of what you want to get out of talking with an expert. One thing about doing interviews is that you only get better at it!

The interview should provide some perks for both of you if planned properly. Just having the opportunity for contact with a "celebrity" can be a thrill in itself, and you might even come up with some significant information (you hope!). Even though the person may be well known, a little extra visibility doesn't hurt. Also, keep in mind that you can elicit superb information from people on your own turf—a colleague, administrator, or perhaps a dean. Don't be reluctant to make the connection.

Before moving ahead, here are some guidelines to assist you. Your prime responsibility is to know something about the person you expect to interview. In other words, *do your homework.* If the individual is quite prominent, be up to date on written works by and about him or her, which can run the gamut from entries in *Who's Who* to a biographical feature story in a magazine.

Unless you are involved in a fairly lengthy profile, your material can probably be obtained via telephone or sometimes through correspondence. If you are interested in just a few responses to questions pertinent to the article, consider sending your queries with a cordial cover letter explaining clearly your purpose. Request permission to quote.

For telephone interviews, write to your subject in advance to elicit his or her go-ahead and to arrange a mutually convenient date and time. With fairly short articles, don't count on in-person interviews unless the people are accessible or suggest meeting with you.

In longer interviews, be sure to have the person's curriculum vitae (c.v.) in advance, whether you're working on a straight profile piece about a well-known figure's life and career, or merely recording a conversation discussing your subject's views on a variety of topics. The c.v. is often a compendium of rich data, containing penetrating clues for you to follow-up on.

As a health professional, you probably use interviewing techniques as part of your everyday work experience with patients, families, employees, and others. Some of the same principles can also apply to authors.

See if the following sounds familiar:

- *Set the right climate for the interview.*

- *Ask questions that will elicit answers.*

- *Know how to listen and pick up important points.*

- *Be sensitive to the person's mood.*

- *Keep person on target if he or she tends to ramble.*

- *Know when to conclude the interview.*

COLLECTING YOUR DATA

When interviewing for an article or book, don't be skittish about asking questions, or thinking that you will impose on the other person. That fear is almost completely unfounded. And if by chance you unwittingly touch upon a sensitive area, your subject will let you know quick enough. In most cases, however, that situation is unlikely to arise if you have done your homework and have developed some insight into the person you will interview.

Another facet of the interviewing process involves your technical skills, which may need some polishing if you intend to use an audio tape recorder. Although a tape recorder is a superb instrument for capturing what people have to say, it has limitations and may intimidate some individuals.

Mishaps do occur, even with the most experienced interviewers running out of or having defective new batteries (always have an extension cord on hand), or experiencing some other problem. A good practice is taking notes even when taping. At the same time, it will enable you to record related observations.

The usefulness of tape recorders, however, can not be overlooked, particularly in the field of oral history. Here, they serve a legitimate purpose although the chief value of a "living history" lies in its final product, the printed transcript. At the same time, taping makes it possible to preserve the voice and remarks of distinguished figures.

Whether or not you intend to record your interviews on audiotape, you should perfect the *act of taking good notes.* Print journalists characterize this process as the true act of writing—a human transaction between two people. Don't be concerned if the person speaks too quickly. Never hesitate to ask him or her to stop for a moment; he or she won't mind because people want to be quoted correctly. In time you will develop your own shorthand and write faster.

When you complete an interview story, it is customary to send a copy, or relevant sections, to the person interviewed. This practice will ensure the accuracy of the material. On shorter articles that include just a few comments of an expert, double check them with your source, preferably during the telephone interview.

When employing the interview process as a means of collecting data for a publishable article, always observe two important standards: *brevity and fair play.* Initially, try to keep the session as brief as possible. Next, present your subject's position accurately, which means never quoting out of context. As a professional, your first obligation is to the individual you interview. Then your "duty" is to your readers, giving them a well presented, factual work.

SUMMARY

The kinds of data—how much or how little—needed to embellish your article depends on the nature of your topic. Since you have already developed the framework with its central message, it's time to forge ahead, eager and willing to nourish your opus with some meaty and relevant content. Put your best sleuthing skills to test and go after the "right stuff!"

LESSON 2

SELF-TEST

Circle the appropriate answer below.   **True   False**

1. Certain types of articles for publication do not lend
   themselves to exploring library sources.   T   F

2. General reference materials contain excellent sources
   for incorporating content into an article.   T   F

3. Periodical indexes and library holdings are your best
   resources for background information on a particular
   topic.   T   F

4. Librarians prefer students and researchers to be more
   self-reliant and search for material on their own.   T   F

5. Identifying key words will expedite a computer search.   T   F

6. If you have the time, you are better off doing a
   computer search than exploring the various indexes and
   library holdings.   T   F

7. It is more preferable to take notes while compiling your
   working bibliography.   T   F

8. The chief criterion for quoting an expert is that the
   person is well known.   T   F

9. Tape recorders should be used whenever possible
   because they will make your work easier.   T   F

10. Your first obligation in an interview-type situation is to
    give your readers a well presented, accurate story.   T   F

Lesson 3

How to Develop Your Article

Now that you have collected your information, the next step is to learn how to use it to produce a rich and interesting article. So far, you have assembled data that include facts, observations, impressions, judgments, generalizations, and other details.

There are several ways to develop a topic in nonfiction prose. You may already know some of these methods, such as *description, narration, exposition,* or *argumentation.* In order to determine which method is most appropriate regarding the content, organization, and style of your paper, you will need to understand each type more fully.

Description

Description—the writer presenting a person, place, or object according to his or her perception—is probably the most familiar method. Description can be used in a variety of ways. For example, you may wish to heighten your reader's understanding of an individual or incident, or provide specific information about something to be explored. Or perhaps you want to convince the audience to buy a certain item. There are times when you may just want to create a feeling or mood in conjunction with one of the other methods of development.

Whatever it is that you are describing, its effectiveness will depend on how precisely you can show how that person, place, or object looked, sounded, felt, tasted, or smelled. You will want to convey a dominant impression—an attitude, image, or feeling that you have about the topic being described.

See if you can identify the dominant impression below:

It was 2 PM when Nurse Shields, carrying a small snack tray, entered Mrs. Gately's darkened room. The only light came from the hall when she opened the patient's door. She saw the blinds drawn and a still figure lying in bed completely covered except for her face. Without expression, Mrs. Gately looked briefly at the nurse and the tray, and then stared straight ahead. Her long gray hair looked uncombed and stringy. When Nurse Shields greeted her and walked toward the bed, Mrs. Gately turned on the other side, covering her face with the bed covers.

You've guessed it! The dominant impression is one of withdrawal. It is reinforced by the darkened room, the expressionless patient, her unkempt hair, rejection of the nurse, and retreating under the bed covers.

A dominant impression can connote fear, serenity, despair, beauty, or any other characteristic, and it may do this alone or in combination with other feelings. When you are able to identify the dominant feeling, it will give unity to your description and help you decide what colorful or vivid details should be added.

Narration

In the most simple terms, narration is story telling. Its purpose is to recount an event (or series of events), usually in chronological order. It enables the reader to relive the event as you have discovered it.

The following excerpt captures the beginnings of the nurse practitioner movement over two decades ago.

In the middle 1960s at the University of Colorado, Loretta Ford, a nurse educator, and a physician colleague, Henry Silver, launched the first demonstration project in the country for the preparation of nurse practitioners. The purposes of that early effort were to improve the health care of children in ambulatory settings by expanding the scope of practice of the registered nurse without altering the nature of nursing, and to explore the nurse's expanded role for program development in collegiate schools of nursing. Although deviations from the project's initial intent occurred, nurse practitioner programs began to appear in several specialty areas. . . . In the spring of 1971, Lucille Kinlein, a registered nurse, hung out her shingle in Suburban College Park, Maryland, to become one of the country's first independent family nurse practitioners.

(Shirley H. Fondiller, The Entry Dilemma)

Your use of chronological progress can be presented in different ways. Rather than arranging events mainly in time sequence, you may wish to stress the most important point first. Then, give the chronological background events, and finally lead into the outcomes of the experience. Another approach would be to begin with your conclusion about the happening and then back track to the unfolding of events leading to that conclusion. Your narrative, in this case, would end with an extension of your earlier introduction.

How you develop the article will reflect your purpose. Ask yourself: "What do I want a narrative format to accomplish that will strengthen the impression I'm trying to make?" Keep in mind that while some narratives operate exclusively on a "what happened" level, others may reflect more depth in trying to show what has been gained or lost during and since a particular period of time. Historians, for example, depict the reasons for social change and influence their readers to explore the values in their own society.

Unlike description, which is viewed as "still," the narrative method connotes action. It will move your story!

Exposition

When used by itself, exposition is a method of development that shows the *how* or *why* something is done. More often, however, it assumes a supporting role in a narration, description, or argument.

Here are some examples of exposition:

- Explaining to a colleague how to prepare a grant proposal.

- Directing a family member to the hospital waiting room.

- Clarifying the discharge plan to a homebound patient.

- Informing your employer of your reasons for accepting a teaching fellowship rather than accepting a promotion to assistant administrator.

Exposition has many forms that every writer should be aware of: *exemplification, process analysis, comparison/contrast, analogy, classification, definition,* and *causal analysis.* These different types can be combined depending on the point you wish to make.

Exemplification.   Through exemplification you provide illustrations, examples, and supporting specific details. The effective use of illustrations is the most important single means of developing ideas. Make certain that they are interesting if you want to develop your point.

Process Analysis.   As another technique, process analysis focuses on the *how* of doing something that involves a series of steps. Some examples might be how to teach patient-controlled anesthesia, how to document nursing practice in a new recording system, or how to do a library computer search.

In process analysis, you present the steps in a clear order, indicating when a certain order is essential. If your reader is not well informed on the topic, you will have to explain in more detail. Also, consider using the second person point of view—the "you"—which suggests a participating audience. If your article is using a case study format, and you are relating a procedure—process analysis could also be used in the first person. In this situation, you would be writing for an observing audience.

Comparison/Contrast.   This form of exposition often produces the best results. Comparison/contrast aims to identify similarities and differences. First, determine your points of comparison and contrast, then decide which points you want to emphasize.

Two basic patterns are evident for organizing your comparison. For example, if you were going to compare health care in the United States with health care in the Peoples Republic of China, you could begin with a sketch of U.S. health care, followed by one of health care in China. Then you would conclude with a section pointing out the similarities and differences revealed by the two descriptions.

Another approach to developing the same topic could be done in this way. Simultaneously describe the number of hospitals in the United States and China, the number and kinds of health personnel, the medical approach to certain health care problems, and so on. Follow with a concluding evaluation of the two systems of health care.

Of the two patterns, the second appears more desirable in that the comparison is explicitly made point by point. At the same time, your readers might find switching back and forth a bit distracting. In such cases, you will have to be the judge of the approach that will make the greater impact in furthering your point. In addition, you can expect to use comparison/contrast with other expository forms, particularly exemplification, analogy, or classification.

Analogy.   This method has some value when you want to compare something that may be unfamiliar or uncommon with something well known or easily understood.

Analogy is a type of comparison but it should never dominate an article or essay. Its purpose is to present a concrete example of a problem without attempting to solve it. In essence, it tries to clarify rather than prove a point.

In using analogy, determine the impression you want to make on your reader about the subject. Next, think of another subject comparable with yours, and find similar areas. Finally, show the comparison between the subjects.

Classification. Classification as a method can be beneficial for arranging a complex set of ideas that share some common feature. Whether it is new immunosuppressant drugs for transplant patients, or diabetes educators in New Mexico that you are trying to "arrange," you will need to study the items to be classified and then choose the basis for the classification. Your selection will depend on what you believe will interest your reader the most.

For example, if you classify diabetes educators for the benefit of Native Americans in New Mexico, you might base your classification on the ability to dispense information, or the ability to obtain compliance with diabetes regimens. Or you might consider another variable. Be certain, however, that all items to be categorized fit into the system.

By using definition and comparison/contrast, you will be able to illustrate in a series of paragraphs the classification options to be covered.

Definition. When you employ definition in an article, you show the specific characteristics that give the term an identity that distinguishes it from other similar terms.

Such concepts as the nursing process or nursing diagnosis may be household words in modern terminology, but not too long ago they were unknown entities. Both terms had to undergo rigorous definition attempting to distinguish nursing process from problem solving (as had been described previously), and nursing diagnosis from medical diagnosis. A flurry of articles soon appeared in the nursing press to define and explain these two terms.

The process of definition is ongoing, particularly since the meaning of concepts vary among individuals and groups. Case management is a good example. It is being implemented across the nation in different institutions and in different ways. Writers, therefore, must be precise about their intent when using definition as a method of development.

The initial step in defining is to identify the *class*—a set or group having at least one common characteristic—to which the term belongs. An obvious example is "shared governance," which fits into the overall category of governance (or perhaps autonomy). Another example, "differentiated practice," would logically be classified under nursing or health care delivery patterns.

After selecting the appropriate class, your next step is to identify the *differentia*, or the specific attributes of the term being defined. The differentia will distinguish the term from others in the same class. For example, primary and team nursing fall within the category of health care delivery patterns, but each modality varies markedly.

Definition is often used with narration, analogy, or other means of developing an article. At some point, you must indicate the term, class, and differentia.

Causal Analysis. This method is another way of saying cause and effect. It can best be developed by analyzing the situation and then discussing the resulting effect. An example familiar to you as a health professional is:

> *Ignoring universal precautions while working in a hospital puts you at risk for H.I.V. infection.*

You would probably have no problem embellishing the above statement with supporting evidence. You could present facts, statistics, illustrations, or case histories through the use of description, narration, or some other approach. Just be sure that when you identify a cause-effect relationship, that one does exist!

Argumentation

What do you think of when you first hear the word "argument?" Two people engrossed in a heated exchange, perhaps shrieking at one another? Sounds logical. But is it?

Realistically, an argument does not have to convey strong emotionalism. Nor must it involve a controversial issue. Furthermore, there may be no opposition to the main point being made.

To argue is simply to give reasons for or against something. When you use argumentation as a method of developing your article, you will experience the act or process of forming reasons, drawing conclusions, and applying them to your discussion. Your main job as a writer is to provide evidence and not rely on common but illogical ways of persuasion.

Argumentation entails inductive reasoning, in which you form a generalization by examining specifics. You then conclude that what is true in specific cases can apply to other similar cases. Here is an example:

> *With the opportunities now available to them in law, medicine, and business, qualified women are opting more for these fields than the traditional*

service professions of teaching, social work, and nursing. (Reason: Studies show that female admissions to medical and law schools have risen sharply, reaching almost 50 percent in many institutions.)

In stating your position, you must convince your reader that your argument is right. You will present your observations, facts, statistics, expert opinions, and other forms of evidence for reaching a sound conclusion.

To make your point effectively, your writing pattern will involve working backward as you review the evidence. Test your reasons on which your case rests to ensure that they support the conclusion. Test your conclusion by asking questions of it. And revise your argument if indicated. Above all, put yourself in your reader's place and you won't go wrong.

Finally, in constructing an argument, try to be objective. You may be quite passionate about your case, but remember that its successful outcome will depend on the supporting evidence regardless of your strong feelings.

What Is Your Point of View?

"I don't know whether to write in the first, second, or third person!" That's a question you may have asked yourself time and time again. And no wonder, there is a great deal of "improper" information being circulated about this concern.

Calm those concerns. There are certain guidelines to follow, with the best guidelines coming directly from the journals themselves. Just thumb through the pages of these publications to see how writers are not only developing their articles but what kind of relationship they establish with their readers and from what perspective. Is the writer involved personally in the experience and, if so, how is it described? Or is the content being presented by an interested but somewhat detached observer?

If the term "point of view" confuses you, stop right there. It does not refer to "viewpoint," which suggests an attitude or a feeling. Rather, the point of view in the writing process is used only in the sense of *person.*

The broadest distinction here is between a personal and impersonal point of view. What distance do you wish to establish between yourself and the audience?

The major determinant for your point of view is your subject matter and your article's purpose. If you are writing about a personal experience, then the natural point of view is from the first person singular. In effect, you are saying to your audience, "I was there. I did so and so. . . ." But there can be exceptions.

As a single author, avoid the use of "We" or the first person plural. It would be unlikely and a bit silly to say: "We walked into the unit to see our patient."

There is a place, however, when to employ "We," as in editorials and whenever the writer is speaking for a group as shown below.

> *When the management team received the report, we concluded that the pilot project could be implemented hospital wide.*

In learning the various methods of development, you already know something about the imperative mood or the use of the second person "You." In such cases, the article addresses readers directly, often showing them a series of steps in a new procedure, treatment protocol, or some other activity.

A writer who wishes to employ the impersonal point of view does not refer to or address the reader in any way. The approach is objective, using the third person, which includes the indefinite or impersonal pronouns (he, she, they, one, it). In this group, try to avoid the word "one" whenever possible because it is often misused and creates a problem.

Objective writing may sometimes appear cold and tedious, and even turn off the audience in some instances. The impersonal style, however, can be humanized by using effective imagery, metaphor, lightness of tone, concreteness, and occasionally humor. Historians and scientists prefer the impersonal point of view, although some writers defer to the use of "we" in reporting their research.

Once you have determined your point of view, try to maintain it since sudden shifts from "I" to "you" to "they" can be distracting. Changes are acceptable, however, but only when your exposition requires it.

Within a single sentence, caution must be exerted in maintaining the same perspective. The following sentence illustrates the shifting point of view from first to second person:

> *A. I was told by my supervisor that* you *should limit the number of Mr. Johnson's visitors.*

Corrected version:

> *B. I was told by my supervisor that* I *should limit the number of Mr. Johnson's visitors.*

SUMMARY

Writers are blessed with a variety of methods and points of view to assist them in perfecting their prose for a publishable article. Study these approaches carefully to ascertain which one should predominate and be consistent with the purposes of your article.

As urged so often, be familiar with the journal market. You can now analyze how different stories are presented and if they follow some of the suggested guidelines or principles contained herein. Be particularly clued in to the needs of your target journal. That includes not just the nature of the articles but how they are treated in their method of delivery and point of view.

As you advance to Lesson 4, you will have arrived at a critical juncture of the writing process. When you successfully complete this step, you will be starting the homestretch of your journey into publishing.

LESSON 3

SELF-TEST

Circle the appropriate answer below.   **True   False**

1. As a method of development, description depends largely
   on the writer's sensory perceptions of the experience
   being described.   T   F

2. The best way to present a narrative is to start from the
   beginning of the situation and proceed chronologically.   T   F

3. Exposition should be used as often as possible by itself.   T   F

4. Process analysis is an effective method that shows how
   to do something in a series of steps.   T   F

5. Because comparison/contrast often produces the best
   possible results, it should not be used with other
   expository forms.   T   F

6. Your reason for using classification to develop your
   article will be based on the need to arrange a complex
   set of ideas with a common feature.   T   F

7. When employing definition, your first step will be to
   identify the special characteristics of the term being
   defined.   T   F

8. In your use of argumentation, your best chance of
   success is the subjectivity of your discussion.   T   F

9. In using casual analysis, the writer analyzes the
   situation and then discusses the effect.   T   F

10. When determining point of view, select the person
    (first, second, or third) that sounds best to you.   T   F

Lesson 4

The Dynamic Duo:
Organizing and Outlining

*T*he most crucial part in preparing an article is not collecting the information or writing the narrative. It is the period in between: *when you decide that what you have gathered is complete and it can be presented.* You are ready for the process of synthesis that will begin with organizing your data and culminate in the writing outline.

Organization is the basis of clarity, and without it the information and ideas in your paper will be unrelated and, therefore, confusing. A long, uninterrupted period is required for the sifting of materials, determining how they relate, and then organizing them into sections.

You already may have formed some ideas in your mind when collecting your data. And as you learned about the different methods of development, you probably shaped your thoughts even further.

Division and *arrangement* represent the two most important steps in organization. You must divide to conquer! The time has come to analyze those precious notes on your index cards, so painstakingly recorded in your earlier search. You will want to ensure the usefulness of each entry for your article. Although it is not unusual to weed out some extraneous information, proceed carefully in this regard.

Decide how you want to categorize your data. Start by jotting down your thoughts, including what you now know about your subject, and then identify the major divisions from the points listed.

When classifying a topic, consider dividing it according to a specific relationship, such as form, function, use, or some other characteristic. Whatever categories you choose, they should be divided into subtopics, depending on the degree of development necessary for the reader to understand your article.

This approach of dividing your subject into major and minor headings enables you to arrange related facts, ideas, or objects in appropriate groupings pointing out their similarities. It will also help you formulate general conclusions.

A question you need to ask yourself is what arrangement will effectively emphasize your major points as well as convince the audience that your topic is valid. All writing should be arranged according to some basis of natural or logical order. For example, if you were describing the growth and development of children up to age five, the natural order would begin with infancy. Here, the approach is inherent in the subject.

Logical order, on the other hand, is imposed by the writer and stems from inference or reason. Keep in mind that the order in which ideas may first occur to you, or how your plan or outline looks at the conclusion of the prewriting process, may not necessarily be the best order for presenting your topic. The chances are, however, that your vibes will be good ones. But a little caution goes a long way.

The Art of Outlining

There is no more effective way to prepare an article than to work from a detailed, sentence outline. The problem with a briefer or more general outline is that most of your thinking has yet to be done, and the constant need to stop and ponder over what to say will make your writing a slow and painful process.

It is true that some experienced writers admit to never or rarely using an outline. In such cases, however, their ideas have probably been well thought out in advance, or they simply write down concepts that form the framework of their paper. These situations are the exception rather than the rule and should not be encouraged for most writers, particularly a novice in the field.

An outline will lay out the plan of your article, giving the fullest statement of your ideas, and showing clearly and explicitly the logical relation of points. Because it forces you to think out your plan so thoroughly beforehand, a well-constructed sentence outline will speed up the actual writing process. You might go so far as to say that the article could even write itself!

THE DYNAMIC DUO: ORGANIZING AND OUTLINING

"How can an outline really help me?" That's a fair question from prospective authors. Quite simply, it will make writing easier and guarantee that it is logical, unified, and properly emphasized. Here's how it can be done.

1. *How can an outline make your writing easier?*

   By ensuring that you've firmed up your thinking and that all the material has been gathered before you begin to write. Also, you should be able to write without interruption.

2. *How does an outline offer a logical, step-by-step method of writing?*

   By listing information in the order in which it will be presented. In addition, it shows graphically the form and progression of your proposed article.

3. *How can an outline ensure that your writing has unity?*

   By allowing you to check relationships between headings. It also helps to recognize and eliminate unnecessary information. Furthermore, it will identify any gaps.

4. *How does an outline help you in achieving proper emphasis in your writing?*

   By checking whether your data are arranged in the order reflecting their relative importance. It will indicate whether your minor points are subordinated properly. Finally, an outline will show whether your statements are properly supported with credible and relevant explanatory information.

Preparing the Plan

Now that you understand the value of a well-developed sentence outline, you're ready to move ahead. Follow these tips about the conventions of outlining.

As you know, every outline consists of an *introduction, body,* and *conclusion*—the same format to be followed in the writing of your article. You will need to replace these three areas with specific and fully developed headings that will be presented in complete sentences.

Your introduction aims to present your main point (topic) and thesis and to stimulate the reader's interest. It will be followed by convincing support in the middle or body. The conclusion or end brings the article to closure by reinforcing your major point.

Review the example in Lesson 1 on the development of a thesis statement. The following illustrates the use of that thesis and the main point in the introductory material of an outline. Note the major and minor headings as well as the grammatical parallelism of the sentences.

I. *INTRODUCTION*

A. Main Point: *Why nurses in a privately funded, nurse-managed teen center, affiliated with a Midwestern university hospital, are key people to provide high-risk adolescents with education and counseling in sexuality and reproductive issues.*

1. *Nurses are viewed as caring people who understand the needs of adolescents.*

2. *Nurses have expertise in communicating information about sexuality and reproductive issues.*

B. Thesis Statement: *The rise of life-threatening illnesses, such as AIDS in inner city adolescents, has demonstrated that such adolescents lack appropriate education or understanding in this area as well as other health problems relating to sexuality and reproduction. Through creative programs, counseling, and referral, nurse practitioners and staff in a nurse-managed teen center have developed a model to reach this population with encouraging results to date.*

1. *The incidence of AIDS among young people is increasing.*

a. *Statistics show a rise in H.I.V. infection among inner city adolescents.*

b. *Educational materials and contraceptive information has had minimal impact.*

2. *Other issues, such as teenage pregnancy, are creating serious health and social problems.*

a. *Demographic data reveal younger adolescents at risk.*

b. *Rejection of prenatal care results in premature births and handicapped infants.*

The above example deals with a complex topic having many facets. Your article may have a narrower focus and, if so, your outline will be less elaborate. As pointed out many times, an article with a less complicated thrust can be just as effective as an article of greater scope requiring considerable detail.

In light of your interest in writing, the following example should be quite informative. Here is a complete outline developed for an article of 1,500 words. Although it is fairly simple due to the nature and length of the paper, the outline will give you some idea of the proper format.

MAKING YOUR SENTENCES COME ALIVE!

I. *INTRODUCTION*

    A. Main Point: *Publishing is an expectation of professional people.*

        1. *Professionals are expected to contribute to the body of knowledge.*

        2. *Professionals have expertise to share.*

    B. Thesis Statement: *Learning proper sentence structure will help writers develop a smooth, facile style to increase their publishing potential.*

        1. *The purpose of writing is to get an idea from one mind to another—clearly, quickly, and economically.*

            a. *Good writing comes only from good thinking.*

            b. *Word power comes from wide and intelligent reading.*

        2. *Nouns and verbs are the building blocks of all writing. (examples)*

II. *BODY*

    A. *A sentence is the setting up of some crucial thought—the subject—and the saying of something about it, the predicate.*

        1. *The subject identifies the topic or theme of the sentence.*

        2. *The predicate says something about the subject, and is the focus of information.*

    B. *A sentence is a self-contained entity that must stand firmly on its own feet.*

        1. *A sentence is complete and thoroughly intelligible.*

            a. *Relative pronouns at the beginning of subordinate clauses are not used as complete sentences. (examples)*

            b. *Relative pronouns are used as complete sentences in the interrogatory sense. (examples)*

        2. *A sentence must be unified containing one dominant theme.*

    C. *According to the kind of clauses they contain, sentences may be classified as simple, compound, complex, or compound-complex.*

1. *Simple sentences are the clearest and most direct. (example)*

2. *Compound sentences enable a rudimentary grouping of statements that help to build up organized thinking. (examples)*

   a. *Compound sentences contain two independent clauses.*

   b. *Compound sentences do not distinguish between the importance of several connected statements.*

3. *Complex sentences indicate the importance of one idea over another. (examples)*

   a. *Complex sentences contain only one independent clause and at least one dependent clause.*

   b. *Complex sentences indicate the central dominant theme of the sentence and what is subordinate to show the exact relationship.*

4. *Compound-complex sentences are used to show coordinated ideas. (examples)*

III. *CONCLUSION*

   A. *A combination of the four categories of sentences helps to provide a smooth, facile writing style.*

   1. *Variety in sentence structure will change the rhythm within a paragraph and keep the reader stimulated.*

   2. *Tips on sentence structure will help to make writing come alive and increase publishing potential.*

   3. *Proper sentence structure will help professionals to increase their publishing potential.*

How to Evaluate Your Outline

When you have completed your outline, you will want to evaluate it for its thoroughness. Check to see if you have done the following:

- Keep your title independent of the text and not as a heading.

- Replace divisions, such as "Introduction," "Body," and "Conclusion," with specific, completely developed headings.
  Ensure that the outline clearly shows the necessary headings, their order, and their relationship.

- Show that all minor (subordinate) headings are logically dependent on the headings immediately superior to them.

- Make sure that the amount of space given to the various headings are proportionate to their relative importance to the subject and the relative amount of space to be given in the completed article.

- Make certain your major and minor headings are grammatically parallel.

- Identify gaps in the outline and eliminate extraneous material.

SUMMARY

Next to developing the right idea for your article, organizing and outlining are the most difficult steps in the writing process. When you have completed the basic work of assembling your material, the time has come to synthesize and arrange it in an orderly fashion.

Through the act of outlining, you will exert control over all your data. It will force you to figure out what you really mean. When completed, this exercise will provide a visual impression that at one glance will enable you to detect any problems. Don't be surprised if you have to fill some gaps and get rid of some kinks. Well-developed headings will tell your story.

Although an outline serves a necessary function, you must remember that it is a means to an end and not an end in itself. As your guide, it may require certain changes or modifications as you move into the writing phase of your article.

LESSON 4
SELF-TEST

Circle the appropriate answer below.	True	False

1. By the time you organize your data, you know exactly what categories or headings will form the basis of your article.　T　F

2. How to classify your data will depend on what your readers need to know and understand about your article.　T　F

3. The main purpose of dividing a subject into major and minor headings is to determine the length of your article.　T　F

4. In arranging your material, the best way to emphasize the major points is according to some basis of natural order.　T　F

5. If you know exactly what to say in your article, an outline is unnecessary.　T　F

6. A well-constructed sentence outline will speed up the writing phase of your article.　T　F

7. A sentence outline will help you to write without interruption.　T　F

8. The two main components of the Introduction are the Main Point and the Thesis Statement.　T　F

9. The more major headings you use, the more substantive your article will be.　T　F

10. Once you have completed your outline, you will have a splendid guide that can be followed without deviation.　T　F

Lesson 5

The Query Letter—
What's It All About?

You may wonder why a letter of query is being introduced at this stage of your lessons. Well, believe it or not, there is a method to this writing "madness." Although no set rule exists as to when to contact an editor about an idea for an article, it is not until you have completed your sentence outline that you can really grasp the scope and significance of your article. Then you will know what to include in your proposal.

Many prospective authors think they have an exciting topic and decide to elicit an editor's interest before doing their homework. All too often, these inquiries are vague and not well thought out. An editor may reject such an idea right off, or suggest that more detail is indicated. There are occasions when an editor will say, "I like your suggestion. Work on it." But don't depend too much on that kind of response. Of course, if you already have completed an article, you can write to an editor at any time, or else send the manuscript with a cover letter.

Delaying a query letter until you finish your outline can be to your advantage because you now will have a substantive plan and a firm hold on your topic. "But what if I've done all this work and no one is interested?" you may ask. A reasonable comment, yes, though it is unjustified. Don't despair.

The chances are that if you have followed the appropriate criteria for focusing on your idea, studied your target journals and their expectations, and performed a thorough search, you will get a positive signal to move ahead on the article. The chief obstacle that may stand in your way is if the journal of choice has recently accepted for publication (but not yet printed) a manuscript on a topic similar to yours. If that occurs, aim quickly for another publication.

One point should be mentioned in regard to approaching journal editors. There are exceptions when you should make contact even though your idea is not fully developed (or if you already have a finished manuscript). As a health professional, no doubt you participate in many conferences, workshops, or seminars. Some of these events, especially national conventions or meetings, usually draw the health press. Although editors and their staff are busy reporting on assignments, they are happy to talk with potential authors, even for a few moments. Don't let this opportunity pass you by. *Always remember, editors need you as much as you need them.* If an editor expresses some interest in your topic, follow through as soon as possible with a letter reminding the person where you met, the nature of your article, and when you expect to complete it.

Why Send a Query Letter?

The answer is probably obvious to you, but a little review may reinforce the advantages of querying editors. You have everything to gain and nothing to lose, assuming you have done your lessons.

Although most editors request letters of inquiry, others have no strong feelings either way. Journal guidelines for authors usually stipulate their preference. Some editors will even respond to telephone queries, but that practice is not recommended for beginning writers.

Your main purpose in writing a letter is to see if a particular editor is looking for the kind of article you are preparing. Not too long ago, the rule was one letter to one editor, but that expectation is no longer valid.

By sending simultaneous query letters, you avoid the delay as well as bother of resubmitting them elsewhere. The only problem in this case (and one with a positive twist!) is if you get the "green light" from two or three journal editors, what do you do? Quite simply, *you accept the assignment from only one editor.* Select the journal that you believe will give your article the most mileage as well as advance you professionally. Be sure to inform the other editors so that they won't expect the article.

Another reason for querying an editor is that it may elicit helpful feedback on how to modify your story or to gear it more toward the journal's audience. Such a response should propel you into action with an all-out effort to expedite your writing! A note of caution, however: An editor's encouragement should not be mistaken for a commitment to publish. Nonetheless, it is a step in the right direction.

What Goes into a Query Letter?

"What kind of stationery should I use to write my query letter?" A silly question? Not at all. Surprisingly, query letters reach editors often in long hand, scrawled on yellow lined paper, personal stationery, note pads, and progress notes! Don't make that mistake.

Above all, never forget that you are a professional. As such, you should know how to write a business letter with all the correct conventions. You will never go wrong with good quality white bond paper—skip the pastels like beige or cream color. If you are affiliated with a college or university, hospital or health care agency, or even have your own company or business, then use that letterhead whether you are an assistant professor, fiscal officer, nurse manager, consultant, or in some other position.

The format of a business letter is as important as the prose and coherent organization that goes into it. Three formats predominate, which you are probably familiar with: *block, modified block,* and *indentation.*

The block style is considered suitable only for letterhead stationery with a printed address. It has become quite popular, with every line beginning at the left margin and containing a single spaced text that is doublespaced between paragraphs. The complimentary closing is parallel to the text.

The modified block format may be used with or without letterhead that has no address. The heading and complimentary closing are aligned just to the right of center. All other elements appear flush with the left margin.

If you are using plain paper, review the indentation pattern in Figure 1. This style places the heading and complimentary closing to the right of center and indents each paragraph five spaces.

Whatever format selected, you can indicate an enclosure or attachment in the left margin at the end of the letter. There is no need to initial the author and typist if you write the letter yourself.

An editor can tell a great deal about a writer from the appearance of the letter. So, know how to present your basic elements—the heading, inside address, salutation, body, and complimentary closing. Figure 1 shows you how to illustrate these properly, including the preferable closing of "Sincerely yours." Some of the more common no-no's that offend editors include signing letters in red ink (it really happens!), or with fanciful endings like "gratefully yours," and using erasable or onionskin paper.

Now that you have the format shaped up, you are ready for the "nuts and bolts" of your query letter. An important tip to help you get the editor's attention is to keep your query letter brief. Editors are busy people, swamped with thousands of letters. When they see a long inquiry from a

Figure 1
Sample Query Letter—Indentation Format

159 Allen Street
Overland Park, Kansas 21063
January 14, 1992

Eleanor B. Martin, M.S., R.N.
Editor
Clinical Digest of Neonatal Nursing
Seven Dupont Circle, NE
Washington, DC 10784

Dear Ms. Martin:

Attached is a summary of a proposed article on new approaches in the nursing care of the newborn with persistent fetal circulation— a health problem with serious implications. As a staff nurse in the special care nursery of a large midwestern hospital, I have worked with these babies for the past three years.

In 1987, I earned a bachelor's degree from the school of nursing, University of Washington (Seattle). Last fall I began part-time study at the University of Kansas, Kansas City, Mo., in the master of science in nursing program. My area of specialization is maternal-child nursing.

Your consideration of my proposal will be appreciated.

Sincerely yours,

Laura Stevenson, R.N.

Attachment

Figure 2
Sample Summary of Proposed Topic

Laura Stevenson
159 Allen Street
Overland Park, Kansas 21063
913/431-6553 (Res.)
816/770-5372 (Bus.)

PROPOSED ARTICLE

"Persistent Fetal Circulation: New Approaches, New Hope"

Through a case study approach, the article will show and compare the effect of modalities in the care of two infants with persistent fetal circulation. Special areas include: nature of the health problem, treatment, nursing monitoring and intervention, interdisciplinary involvement, and family participation.

Action photos are available.

Length of article: 2000 words.

prospective author, their first tendency is to put it aside or just scan the beginning.

An effective approach, and most editors seem to like the idea, is attaching a summary of your proposed idea to the query letter. In this way, you're bound to get a fair shake.

When you decide on your target journals(s), the first step is to get the correct name of the person to contact, generally the editor or editor-in-chief, or as in the case of *Nursing*, the clinical director. The proper place to locate the information is in the staff box of the most recent issue. Looking it up in a journal six months to a year old can be counter-productive.

Since editors tend to be mobile, you may find your inquiry reaching someone who left months (sometimes years) earlier. What does that tell the present editor? That you are not on the ball or you're not familiar with the journal.

Other resources, such as directories published in books and magazines, often carry data about editorial staff and journal requirements. Such guides can be quite useful but the names of editors, if listed, could be old hat by the time the publication comes out.

The staff box appears in the beginning of a journal, usually in the first, two, or three pages. Sometimes, it has a heading of "Editorial Staff," although more likely it starts with the editor's name followed by the supporting staff—associate editors, managing editor, editorial assistants, and so on. The names of editorial advisors may also be in the staff box, but often they are listed separately. In Lesson 9, you will learn more about the role of journal editorial boards and/or advisory committees.

At the bottom of the staff box, or on the same page, you may find information about where to send your query letter or manuscript. Guidelines for authors also give details. If you have questions, call the journal directly.

When addressing your letter, look carefully at the spelling of the editor's name and the credentials used. Even though it is considered better form to place academic degrees before professional titles, such as Alice Porter, MS, RN, you will see the opposite order in some journals. The latter is not viewed as incorrect, but the other is preferable according to the "experts" (see the style guides of the *New York Times* and *Associated Press*). Be sure, however, to follow the way the name and title appear in the journal.

Finally, a note of caution. If you query more than one editor, make sure the right letter goes into the right envelope! This point may seem academic, but unfortunately mistakes occur with both letters of inquiry and manuscripts (which should only be sent to one journal anyway). No need to comment on the implications. Such carelessness can turn off an editor.

THE QUERY LETTER—WHAT'S IT ALL ABOUT?

There is no rule that says a procedure must always be done in a particular way to be effective. Yet, when it comes to a query letter, one thing is certain. Most editors do not want long, wordy letters. Either send one letter making it succinct, or follow the format in Figures 1 and 2 in which your summary proposal is on a separate sheet. Here is appropriate content to be included with the letter using the latter approach:

- Title and nature/central message of proposed article.

- Rationale for attracting the readership.

- Your qualifications to write the article (experience, education).

- Other information—if you have published recently, or if there are contributing authors.

If you are well into your paper, inform the editor and indicate when you expect to complete it. Or, if you have already completed the manuscript, either mention this or send the work with a cover letter.

Your query letter not only gives some idea of your background, but provides clues about your ability to express yourself. Although you want to grab that editor's interest at the beginning, play it straight. Start right off with the central message of your article and your attached proposal will do the rest.

In the summary that defines your proposed topic, keep the length to 75 words (or less) unless the guidelines for authors stipulate otherwise. On the sheet, include your name and address, and also your telephone number where you can be reached during the day. On occasion, journal editors have been known to phone potential authors when a novel or unusual idea excites them. Also, you never know when the story you are suggesting may be just what an editor has been seeking for an upcoming issue. What could be more motivating than a go-ahead like that!

Using Figures 1 and 2 as illustrations, include the following points in your summary proposal:

- Title of article.

- Nature of article.

- Major points or areas to be covered.

- Proposed length (words or pages typed double space).

- Photos, charts, tables, or other visuals.

Following Through on Query Letters

How long should it take an editor to answer a query letter? Although it is possible that you may receive a postcard acknowledging your inquiry or even a letter within a few weeks, don't be alarmed if you don't hear right away.

Editors may be out of town (or out of the country) at conventions or conferences, on vacation, or even be involved in in-house meetings. They also may want to share your letter with staff or advisors for an appraisal of your topic. Then again, they could be bogged down with other correspondence waiting to be addressed.

How quickly editors respond depends on their priorities. If no word is forthcoming in a month's time, by all means write (rather than telephone) to the journal again, but always be cordial. You could use the following example as a guide.

Dear Ms. Porter:

I wonder if you reached any conclusion about the article I proposed in my letter of January 5, 1992. Enclosed is a copy of my summary proposal that I sent with the letter.

Your comments will be appreciated.

Sincerely yours,

Margaret Dunlap, M.A.

O.T.R.

Encl.

There is always the possibility that the original letter was lost or mislaid or the proposal detached. Your second query should elicit a fairly prompt reply.

When editors acknowledge query letters, they can respond in various ways. You need to know why most suggested topics are rejected. Any concern you may have should be minimal, however, because your topic has been based on sound criteria, familiarity with your target journal and its guidelines, and a solid outline.

THE QUERY LETTER—WHAT'S IT ALL ABOUT?

Here are the more common reasons for rejecting a topic:

- It seems to say nothing new.

- It is overworked in the literature.

- It has no significance or contemporary relevance.

- It is too far out—limited appeal.

- It is not suitable for this journal.

- Similar article has been accepted by editor.

When submitting a letter of inquiry, it is difficult to predict an editor's reaction. What one editor may like about your proposal, another may not. In cases where two journals have similar audiences, the decision rests on priorities and needs. Perhaps your topic will be especially timely, fitting in with a thematic issue being planned for the near future.

If the editor approves your idea, you may be given carte blance to move ahead with the article. Or there may be suggestions to alter the focus. When changes appear too drastic, requiring a substantive rewrite of your outline, you will have to decide whether to invest in the effort. "Do I have the expertise for the proposed new slant?" "Should I query another journal about my original idea?" Only you can respond to these questions.

You probably will have mixed feelings. After all, you have invested a lot of energy into your topic. At the same time, the editor has presented you with a challenge and if you think that you're up to it, then "bite the bullet." Such perseverance often pays off, and if the editor accepts your article for publication, you will have made an important new contact in the editorial world.

When interest is expressed in your proposed topic, send the editor pronto a short letter of intent indicating that you are writing the article and plan to complete it within a certain time. Don't hem yourself in, however, with a specific date because you will find yourself in a bind. The act of writing and especially rewriting takes longer than you think. Your goal is to submit a finished product—a polished manuscript. So don't wait. Work at a steady pace.

In some situations, an editor will request a manuscript by a certain date. If that expectation is realistic for you, then follow through. If not, you may want to telephone the editor directly explaining your reasons for a short delay. Unless they have a set deadline to meet, editors are quite understanding when authors need more time. Therefore, don't be reluctant. It is better to be candid than to make a commitment you can't keep.

SUMMARY

No matter how many query letters you send simultaneously, their aim is to elicit interest in your potential article. You are not bound by them to any editor when merely making an inquiry. If you confirm, however, that the completed manuscript will be submitted to a particular journal, you are obligated to send it to that journal—until you know its status.

When you are in the process of developing your story, querying editors will save you time and effort. Most of all, it will put you on the right track to a marketable article.

LESSON 5
SELF-TEST

Circle the appropriate answer below.   **True   False**

1. Sending a query letter early in the writing process is the best time to elicit a positive response from an editor.   T   F

2. Most editors would rather receive manuscripts than query letters.   T   F

3. If you get a positive response to three query letters, confirm with the three editors to ensure your chances of acceptance of the finished article.   T   F

4. A good reason for querying an editor is to get helpful feedback.   T   F

5. Writing a letter in long hand is acceptable if written neatly.   T   F

6. Any format for a business letter can be used if it is typed neatly.   T   F

7. Attaching to the query letter a summary of your proposed topic can be an effective way to catch the editor's attention.   T   F

8. If you don't know the editor's name, it is acceptable to address your query letter to just the Editor.   T   F

9. A month is a reasonable length of time to wait for a response to your query letter.   T   F

10. If an editor encourages you to go ahead with your article, you should give a date when you expect to complete it.   T   F

Lesson 6

The "Catchy" Lead to Logical Conclusion

With a well-defined outline in hand, you are ready to explore in more detail the organizing framework of your article. Three becomes the magic number with the introduction, body of the paper, and its conclusion. As you know, the beginning sets forth your thesis whereas the middle part amplifies and provides convincing support for your main point. Finally, the end lets the reader know he or she has arrived and your mission has been accomplished.

A strong opening or lead is important to the success of your article because it will introduce the central theme and entice the reader into the text. With the number of health care journals flooding the market, and the limited time health professionals have to keep up with them, people are becoming highly selective in what they read. What do *you* first look for in perusing a journal? Promos on the cover? The table of contents to scan the titles or the names of authors? Or perhaps you just flip through the pages to see what catches your eye.

The choice of a particular article and whether it will succeed in sustaining audience interest depends to a large extent on the introduction. Readers are fidgety people who will move on to the next piece unless you "grab" them from the beginning. The first sentence has some real work to do because it must tug the reader into the second and remaining sentences in the opening paragraph. Once you've hooked your reader, you can consider it a major coup but only because you are promising that the best is yet to be.

Good and Bad Leads: What's the Difference?

Articles appearing in health care publications reflect leads of all sizes and shapes, with many good and others not so good! In time, you will get to know the difference. Some are dull and turn the audience off at the outset. This is unfortunate because the body of the story may have exciting new material. The responsibility lies with both author and editor, but editorial referees or reviewers also have a say in the presentation of an article. Editors who are savvy about the importance of interesting leads revise them as needed.

What are some of the pitfalls to avoid in working on your introductory statement? It will be useful to be aware of the more common ones before describing what makes a good opening. Here are some pointers:

1. *Overworked Introduction.* Do not start with a dictionary definition. Instead, state the term in your own words and what it means to you.

   Poor. Webster states that *quality* means . . . .

   Improved. A unique new standards tool recently implemented in a southeastern community hospital has markedly influenced the *quality* of care given by new graduates.

2. *Superfluous Introduction.* Do not begin with the phrase—"The purpose of this article is . . . ." This statement appears repeatedly in journals and detracts from the article.

   Poor. The purpose of this article is to show that case management can be a cost-effective approach in patient care.

   Improved. Case management can be a cost-effective approach in patient care.

3. *Trite Introduction.* Avoid an opening that asserts something commonly known.

   Poor. From the beginning of time, stroke has been a major health problem.

   Improved. Advanced modalities in the treatment of stroke patients are giving new hope to them and their families.

Now that you know some of the *nays* in beginning an article, it's time to accentuate the *yays* and show all the good ways and even the fun you can have in creating your own thing. Yes, developing your introduction will be a terrific test of your ingenuity.

Before starting, however, keep in mind that the lead does not have to be firmed up before continuing with the rest of the paper. Some writers hold off on the introductory paragraph until *after* completing the first draft. At that point, you may have a better idea of the kind of opening strategy that will best fit the work. It is also possible that in reviewing your draft, you may find the lead buried in the third, fourth, or some other paragraph. So, don't belabor the opening too much unless you are already set on a super beginning.

Follow the following suggestions and you're bound to come up with the right opening.

Lead with Your Thesis Statement. A well-developed thesis reveals your central message right away. Recall the thesis statement illustrated in Lessons 1 and 4:

> *The rise of life-threatening illnesses such as AIDS in adolescents has demonstrated their lack of education or understanding in this area as well as other health problems related to sexuality and reproduction. Through creative programs, counseling, and referral, nurse practitioners and staff in a nurse-managed teen center have developed a model to reach this population with encouraging results to date.*

The above thesis comprises the entire introductory paragraph. Its approach is forthright, showing exactly what the article is about—the development of a model involving a special population. As a lead, it may appear cut and dried, but the topic is timely and presented clearly. The chances are that it will draw readers.

Lead with a Scene Stealer. By depicting a scene that will appeal to the reader's senses as well as helping the reader get hold of your topic, you can gradually lead into your thesis. Joyce Zerwekh (1991) illustrates this point in her article, "True Detectives: Tales from Public Health Nursing," which appeared in the *American Journal of Nursing.* See if you agree.

> *You walk into the house and see two babies in a perfectly clean room, with only one toy—a rattle. In another room, you find an extremely attentive mother who nevertheless feels she is going crazy. Or you visit a woman who you suspect is trying to kill herself by neglecting her ulcer. Or you meet a father who has strung Christmas lights around his baby's crib.*

Pretty graphic examples, aren't they, but you get the picture. The author's next paragraph begins with: *The public health nurse is a detective looking for clues.* The body of the article develops this point substantively through the use of description and narration primarily.

Lead with a Quotation. Some editors reject quotations as openings because they often suggest nothing new. At the same time, this method can stimulate humor or provide a beginning framework for an article. Introducing a story with such overworked phrases as the Great Bard's "To Be or Not to Be . . ." should be avoided whenever possible.

In the *Nursing Outlook* article, "Endowed Chairs in Nursing," by Joyce Fitzpatrick (1991), the author prefaces the piece with a familiar Nightingale quote citing nursing as the "finest of arts." In this case, the excerpt seems acceptable in light of the transition to the opening paragraph:

> *Perhaps if Florence were alive today, she would conclude as we have, that not only is nursing the finest art, but also an important scientific scholarly enterprise. Our focus on an endowed chair in nursing is a symbol of our advancements within the great universities in our nation, for an endowed chair is the highest academic position to which a faculty member can be appointed.*

Lead with a Question. A plausible or provocative question as an opener can almost immediately clue in the reader to the gist of the article. Here is an example.

> *Is today's MBA obsolete tomorrow? A fair question for health care managers. Only a few years ago, thousands were flocking to college campuses for that business credential guaranteeing lifetime job security. But no more. Technology is taking over and in a decade the irreplaceable MBA will be a thing of the past.*

The above paragraph introduces the topic with an intriguing question. It has a futuristic twist that conjures up a number of issues. The author has sounded a challenge, reaching the reader at his or her highest peak. When you begin with a question, it should have an element of surprise. Otherwise, the lead sounds mundane and you may lose your audience.

Lead with an Anecdote. A short narrative chronicling of an incident can be highly effective in capturing a reader's attention. In "Coping with Fears of

Caring for HIV-Positive Patients," Marshelle Thobaben (1991) presents the following introduction in the *Home Healthcare Nurse* article:

> *In the coffee room recently a group of home health nurses were discussing their fears of caring for HIV-positive patients. . . . "I am afraid I will stick my finger with a contaminated needle and die from AIDS." "Not enough is known about the disease. The government has been reluctant to protect health professionals." "I feel anxious and stressed every time I have to draw blood from an HIV-positive patient. . . . My husband wants me to quit my job. He's afraid I'll become infected."*

This excerpt from the author's introduction presents in anecdotal format the concerns of several home health nurses caring for HIV-positive patients. The reader can empathize with this human problem. Fears are verbalized, and there is the expectation from the title and lead that the article will have some answers.

Lead with an Example.   When writers begin with one or more examples, they are showing rather than telling what is to come. In her *Nursing 89* article, "A New Approach to Better Medication Compliance," Jo Gibson (1989) states her message early on:

> *Barbara Mason, an epileptic patient, hasn't had a seizure in 5 months. So she's decided not to take Dilantin anymore.*

> *Thomas Peiffer, who has congestive heart failure, hasn't seen his grandchildren in months. Tomorrow they're coming to visit. He doesn't want to be embarrassed by making frequent trips to the bathroom, so he's stopped taking his Lasix.*

> *Wanda Jamison is supposed to take one digoxin tablet daily. But whenever she feels a heart palpitation, she takes an extra one.*

The reader identifies with the above examples which are realistic. The fact that the author has used complete names enhances the believability of the situation. Nothing is more dehumanizing than labeling hypothetical people as Mr. J. or L. B.

After opening the article with illustrations, the author leads the audience to her main point, summing up the dangers of noncompliance. From the outset, she provides an answer to the problem identified: a model for a self-medication program.

Leading with an example is also an excellent way to begin an article when using the case method approach. The introduction sets the tone from the start, making it easier for the reader to follow the patient or central person throughout the story to its conclusion.

Whatever lead you may decide to pursue in your article, make sure it is fresh, fairly brief, and above all interesting. Humor, surprise, and novelty are all eye-catchers. Don't get too caught up with the jargon of your trade. Learn how to make that proper transition from reporting clinical or academic notes to reporting in a professional journal. Take a good topic, develop it with ease and simplicity, and your reward will be a captive audience!

The Body of the Article—What It Needs

Whether you have the lead paragraph finalized, or are still deliberating over the best way to introduce your topic, you can still move ahead and develop the body of your article. The middle section provides the evidence needed to persuade the reader of what you are saying. This is the "meat" of your opus, in which you will build on the who, what, why, how, when, and where of your thesis.

At this stage, your outline becomes an indispensable resource because it shows the sequential development of the paper. Use this guide plus your notes and annotated bibliography as supporting information to embellish your topic. You now need to convert all those facts, opinions, explanations, statistics, and other material into practical but eloquent prose that will give the article a vitality as well as credibility.

The methods of development that you learned about in Lesson 4 will assume great import. You may wish to review this lesson to reinforce your original selection or possibly consider other options. Whether you choose description, narration, exposition, or argumentation, you will be ready to combine style with substance. This is a formidable challenge, but you will be up to it!

Leading to a Logical Conclusion

As you put the finishing touches on the middle part of your article, you have reached a pivotal point in the writing process. You are ready to move into the concluding phase—your last opportunity to provide the reader with a way of reviewing the work as a whole. Your conclusion can be written as a separate paragraph or tacked on to the body of the paper. However presented, it should bring your story to a measured stop so that the audience is not left dangling in the air.

THE "CATCHY" LEAD TO LOGICAL CONCLUSION

Unless indicated in a journal's guidelines, try to avoid using the heading of "Conclusion" (except in reports of studies). If you need to make a transition from the previous section, use a heading that encompasses the salient points in the concluding paragraph.

A number of options are available in determining the kind of ending that best reflects the purpose of the story as well as the thesis set forth. The summary is the most simple and often the best means to meet this aim. It works particularly well in argumentative and expository writing, in which the author taps the reader's recall of the thesis statement and reinforces the supporting main points.

In Thobaben's article, mentioned previously, the author brings the ending to a logical close in this way:

> *In summary, staff fears about working with HIV-positive patients constitute a serious problem that has the potential of interfering with the provision of quality care. It is a joint responsibility of the agency and the staff to solve the problems so that HIV-positive patients are not mistreated and the staff feels supported and safe in caring for them.*

In another article cited, Zerwekh uses a summary statement to wrap up her story about public health nurses as "true detectives." She emphasizes how nurses, through their detecting skills, have created solutions to help the patients described. An anecdotal account of a real situation illustrates this point and effectively concludes the piece.

Before employing the summary ending, check your target journal(s) to see how conclusions are presented in the articles. Although most editors do not object to the use of a summary, there may be one or two who prefer other approaches. Articles also may conclude with a prediction, question, quotation, recommendation, or a combination of these methods. Using a prediction has merit in a narrative or discussion that stresses cause and effect.

If you decide to end with a question, you are allowing the audience to make its own predictions and form its own conclusions. This approach involves readers in the logical process of argument. When you raise a question in your final paragraph, you can hope to influence them in one of three ways: (1) those opposing your views will have at least allowed themselves to reconsider the issue; (2) those previously uncertain may decide to agree with you; or (3) those who already support your views will hold them more strongly.

Another method, that of concluding with a quotation, allows you to cite the opinion of an expert in the area discussed in your article. Keep such a quote brief, however, and make sure it is relevant. If it sounds contrived, you will hurt all the good work done on the article and let your reader down. When in doubt, rethink your ending.

Some authors conclude with recommendations when they want to emphasize action to be taken. Reports of research often include suggestions for replication or for further studies.

No author has to be limited to one choice in considering how to conclude an article. Some topics lend themselves to a combination of the methods described. Whatever your preference, remember that devising an effective conclusion will depend on your response to two basic questions: "Who is my audience and what kind of ending will draw readers to my way of thinking?"

WRITING UP STUDIES—WHAT JOURNALS WANT

A primer on writing would be incomplete without discussing the organizing features of articles describing research conducted by health professionals. Indications are that the publishing of studies no longer falls within the exclusive bailiwick of the scientific or research journals. Instead, some publications that have focused mainly on the how-to type of article in the past are beginning to fill their pages with reams of studies.

Although there is a place for investigations in such journals, the audience may be shortchanged when study reports take precedent over other types of articles. Guidelines for authors spell out what editors are seeking, and most of them give authors a variety of options consistent with their journal's purpose. Articles on studies may be encouraged, but manuscripts reflecting new programs, patterns of care, educational innovations, and so on should indeed rate a high priority.

The trend toward publishing more research pieces is not surprising in light of the current push in that direction among the health disciplines. Scientific inquiry is essential to the survival of any learned profession. If you want to write about a study that you conducted or participated in, look over the different journals to determine the most appropriate one for your topic. Keep in mind that your research must be fairly recent as well as completed (unless it is a longitudinal investigation).

The Research Journal: A Set Format

In journals devoted primarily to research, the editor usually stipulates a circumscribed format that follows the scientific process. Specific directions are available on the preparation of the abstract that precedes the report. The article begins with an *introduction*, which defines the problem to be explored. Next comes the *literature review, method, results,* and *discussion*. A *conclusion* finalizing the report may suggest other studies to be undertaken.

As you know there are all types of research. In clinical investigations, the goal is to improve practice. Therefore, you must describe it clearly as well as credibly or no one in the practice area will apply your findings. The two greatest barriers to the use of research by clinicians relate to the characteristics of the setting and the way the study is presented. As a general tip, try to shift the emphasis away from the theoretical and methodological considerations. Instead, focus on the instrument, intervention, and results, showing through discussion their usefulness and feasibility.

Although the organizing pattern appears similar in most research publications, some vary the style from article to article. Don't be surprised if you see some steps combined to allow for conciseness. Also, not all research journals report only studies since some carry features on theory, methodology, and other topics of audience interest.

Studies in Non-Research Journals

Non-research journals that publish studies from time to time may use a less formal outline in describing the work. When headings are used, they often indicate the gist of the content that follows.

No matter how small or simple a study may be, your design, method, and implementation must be sound. Your report will be judged by a panel of experts who critique all manuscripts with the potential for publication. In Lesson 9, you will learn how these editorial referees operate.

A study that is informative and well expressed should excite an audience. In many cases, however, readers tend to shun research articles because of the technical and tedious writing, which is intensified by an overdependence on the passive voice. If your bent is toward writing up some investigation that you have been involved in, be thorough, brief, and summarize whenever necessary. Above all, cultivate those active verbs!

SUMMARY

The importance of a good introduction cannot be overstated. If it does its job correctly, the audience will be sufficiently coaxed to read on. The momentum, however, must be sustained throughout, meaning that the body of the article will have to live up to the expectations of the lead with informative supporting material. That will depend on the evidence itself and the writer's skill in conveying the article's message through an effective method of development. The conclusion will restate the thesis and sum up the major points. Readers are thus able to see the work as a whole.

In the research realm, the increased output of studies appearing in the journal literature seems to reflect the larger trend of investigations underway in the health care community. Non-research publications have joined the movement and many are publishing reports of studies. As with other kinds of articles, certain principles of good writing must be followed whether you are into clinical, educational, managerial or some other type of research.

LESSON 6
SELF-TEST

Circle the appropriate answer below.   **True   False**

1. A published article shows that the lead is good and will
   be read.   T   F

2. Your lead does not have to be firmed up before getting
   into the body of the article.   T   F

3. You don't have to get into the thrust of your article
   until you begin the middle section.   T   F

4. A familiar quotation is an excellent way to begin an
   article.   T   F

5. Readers like an example at the beginning because they
   can identify with it.   T   F

6. How well you develop the body of the article will depend
   on the method you use.   T   F

7. The conclusion is less important than the introduction
   or body of the article.   T   F

8. A conclusion should always be set off in a separate
   paragraph.   T   F

9. Non-research journals are overstressing reports of
   studies in lieu of other types of articles.   T   F

10. Studies published in non-research journals should follow
    the typical research format.   T   F

Lesson 7

The Moment of Truth: Your First Draft

As you begin the writing phase of your article, never forget that your basic purpose is to communicate. You may have the best topic in the world but if your biggest block is expressing yourself, you may be in trouble. So far, you have gone through all the preparatory steps in the writing process. Now, the day of reckoning has come and you must sit down at your typewriter, computer, or however you work best, to launch that first draft.

Before starting, however, it will help as well as reassure you to review some of the principles of good writing. By following these simple rules, you will be able to move more easily through the various revisions of your paper to completion.

THE ART OF SELF-EXPRESSION

David Lambuth (1964), Dartmouth's great English professor of the 1920s and nurturer of a whole host of distinguished American authors, once said, "When you write, make a picture with nouns. And make that picture move with verbs."

Nouns and verbs are indeed the building blocks of all writing. When your nouns are strong, you don't need to dress them up with adjectives.

When your verbs are busy doing and making something, they will give vitality to the work as well as enhance the power of your language.

Keep in mind that your writing to be effective must be set down in simple and natural speech and revised later in accordance with good usage. Beef up your word power by wide and intelligent reading.

A person who thinks clearly will write clearly. Conversely, someone whose thinking is vague or lazy will end up with a badly constructed paper. Obscurity is not profundity!

Here's something that everyone has experienced. How many times have you read an article (or even a sentence or paragraph) one, two, or three times, and you still can't comprehend the meaning? Well, don't chastise yourself. The fault is neither in the stars nor in you. The burden falls squarely on those authors who, for whatever reason, have not conveyed clearly what they want to say. Don't let that happen to you.

Streamlining Your Sentences

Glance over the outline, "Making Your Sentences Come Alive," which appears on pages 43–44 in Lesson 4. Then see how the following narrative describes some (but not all) of the points made in the supporting sentences. The headings are consistent with the thesis statement: *Learning proper sentence structure will help writers develop a smooth, facile style to increase their publishing potential.*

A sentence is essentially the setting up of some central thought—the *subject*—and the saying of something about it—the *predicate*. While the subject identifies the topic or theme of the sentence, which is being discussed, the predicate says something about the subject and is the focus of information. A sentence is the simplest form in which a complete and independent statement of fact can be made. Therefore, it becomes the unit of all logical thinking.

As a self-contained entity, your sentence must stand firmly on its own feet. If the statement is not complete and thus not thoroughly intelligible, the thought you may be trying to express will be broken and imperfect. This is why it would be unwise for you to write subordinate clauses, such as those beginning with the relative pronouns *who, which, that,* the conjunction *though,* or the adverb *where* as though they were complete sentences. To illustrate:

> *Who reported the weekend accident*
>
> *Which she discarded*
>
> *Though he had seen the patient before*
>
> *Where he had been one time*

It is another matter, however, to use *who, which, and where* in the interrogative sense such as *Who reported the weekend accident?*

In addition to being complete, a sentence must be unified. Your readers will expect a sentence to express just one dominant thought, and if it does otherwise they will feel misled. When a sentence contains two or more distinctly separate statements, it lacks unity and should be broken up into two more statements.

All too often, beginning writers have a proclivity for connecting disparate thoughts with the conjunction *and.* Try to avoid this pitfall. If you find your sentence is not going well, stop and ask yourself: "What is it I am really talking about?" Then determine your central idea and put it down as the subject of the sentence. The remaining thought should flow more easily.

According to the kind of clauses they contain, sentences may be classified as *simple, compound, complex,* or *compound-complex.* Simple sentences are the clearest and most direct, but when used all the time they are disjointed and monotonous. They also will tend to make your writing seem choppy. Because they stand alone and carry equal weight with every other sentence, they fail to build up a thought or a series of thoughts.

A simple sentence has only one independent clause and no dependent clauses. By accumulating phrases it may be quite long.

Here is a simple sentence with only a subject and its verb:

She practiced.

Here is a simple sentence with more embellishment:

The physical therapist showed her patient some new exercises.

Compound sentences enable a rudimentary grouping of statements that help to build up organized thinking. They do not make it possible, however, to distinguish clearly between the importance of the several connected statements. As a result, your sentence becomes stringy.

A compound sentence contains at least two independent clauses and should be used only when you want to give equal emphasis to two related ideas. The clauses are usually joined by a comma and a conjunction (*and* or *but*) or by a semicolon. Also, you can use compound sentences when attempting to express coordinate ideas in comparison, contrast, or balance. See below:

1. *You take the day shift, and I'll take the night shift.*

2. *The nursery was chilly, but it heated up after the nurse called maintenance.*

3. *The staff initiated case management; it began with an orthopaedic critical pathway.*

In shifting to complex sentences, you should know that they alone indicate the importance of one idea over another. They also give a sense of the interrelatedness of ideas essential to accurate thinking. Learn to use complex sentences because they will help to stylize your article. They contain only one independent clause and at least one dependent clause:

When David S. Trufant became dean, he drew faculty from all over the country. (Dependent clause: When . . . dean; independent clause: He . . . country)

You will clarify your thoughts only when you have learned to select almost unconsciously the central, dominant theme of your sentence, and to group around it in varying degrees of emphasis:

Loretta Devon's opportunities had been limited; she studied hard to earn the clinical doctorate; she graduated at the top of her class.

The statements above are presented clearly, but they fail to indicate exactly what the writer had in mind. What do you think is the dominant thought in the sentence? What should be subordinated?

The important idea here is that in spite of limited opportunities, Loretta Devon succeeded because she studied hard. If you subordinate properly, you will not only state all of the original ideas but also bring out their exact relationship. Please note:

Although Loretta Devon's opportunities had been limited, she graduated at the top of her class because she studied hard to earn a clinical doctorate.

Finally, the compound-complex sentence is used when you want to show coordinate ideas, either or both of which are qualified. It consists of one or more dependent clauses and two or more independent clauses. See this example:

When the clinical specialist handed in his clinical exam (dependent clause), *he looked anxious* (independent clause), *but he left the room confidently.* (independent clause)

In an article, you can mix the four categories of sentences appropriately as you write and revise a paragraph. The variety that you show in your sentences will change the rhythm within the paragraph as well as keep your readers stimulated by your prose. Furthermore, however you classify them, your sentences should be written clearly, concisely, and carefully. Don't become a captive of the unwieldy or run-on sentence. No one said it better than Shakespeare: "Brevity is the soul of wit!"

Pampering Your Paragraphs

Like sentences, paragraphs need some coddling. The topic sentence introduces the subject and main thought. Although generally the topic sentence initiates the lead paragraph, it can be placed in other positions depending on the emphasis you wish to achieve. When all the sentences provide convincing support for the topic sentence, your paragraphs will have unity. Nothing is more frustrating to readers when succeeding sentences appear unrelated. This is a serious limitation of the paper showing a lack of development of the paragraph's main idea. So, make sure your sentences are logically and fully connected.

"How long should my paragraphs be?" you may wonder. In at least four or five sentences, you should be able to persuade the audience of the validity of your main points. If the paragraphs are too brief or too long, your readers will get bored or distracted. When you have additional information on a particular topic, start another paragraph.

To move smoothly from one thought to another, make the necessary transition. Sometimes, you can make the change with only a single word or phrase, such as "On the other hand," "In view of the above," or "Although." Transitions are like bridges, connecting one idea with another so that readers can see the relationship. When you want to separate, summarize, compare or contrast, or emphasize certain areas, the transitional paragraph will meet that need.

Combining Style and Substance

Style and substance are the backbone of a successful article. The substance part evolves from your efforts as a responsible and thorough sleuth tracking down a worthy topic. Your writing style stems in part from an inherent creativity but it is a skill nourished by good readings and practice of your craft.

Who hasn't heard of the Strunk and White (1978) little classic, *The Elements of Style?* But another dandy resource is Karen E. Gordon's (1984) *The Transitive Vampire,* a highly imaginative handbook of grammar targeted for "the innocent, the eager, and the doomed." You will love it!

For other sources on composition and writing, study the bibliography at the end of the workbook. Also, Appendix A illustrates some of the do's and don'ts of modern usage. Also, some illustrations of the do's and don'ts of modern usage are shown on pages 169–172.

CREATING A WRITING ENVIRONMENT

You are almost ready for that first draft, but not quite. Some important preliminary work is yet to be done. As with all writers, you will need to develop your own writing lifestyle. What this means is establishing a regimen that will foster the right climate for getting on with your opus as quickly as possible.

The days of procrastination are over. Self-deception as the real destroyer of writing time is out and self-discipline is in. Excuses such as there being no time to write while holding a job will fall on unsympathetic ears, since most authors are fully employed. They have earned their glory through boldness and determination. And so will you.

Set a Writing Schedule

In initiating a working-writing schedule, harness yourself and stick to it. Don't wait until the spirit moves you because there always will be peak periods and down periods. Just keep at it.

Sure you are human and will do anything to delay the task. Besides, isn't it the perfect time to clean the tropical fish tank, or take on some other long overdue chore? Or maybe you can't resist saying no this one time to a friend with an extra ticket for a great matinee. Instead of buckling down to the "writing board," you will think of scads of things you would rather do— cycling in the park, skiing on the slopes, or sailing on the seas. Or maybe you should just wait for a rainy day.

Humbug! No one will print your alibi. So face it, the moment of truth is approaching. Why not follow the advice of Commander Perry when he wanted to get to the North Pole: "Find a way or make one."

Since you know yourself better than anyone, *you* will have to decide on the best time to do your writing. A daily routine of rising early in the morning before going to your regular job may be just your thing. You would be surprised how much can be accomplished in a couple of hours before the rest of the household awakens. If you don't have a family, the potential for interruptions is even less.

Many writers adhere to this pattern religiously and succeed in publishing articles and books one after another. But if getting up in the morning's wee hours is not for you, then look into other options. Perhaps you prefer weekends, setting aside a Saturday and/or Sunday, or even some week nights.

Two cardinal rules must be followed when determining your writing time: (1) be consistent in the schedule you select and (2) be alert and fresh. Nothing dulls the creative processes more than fatigue, which will ultimately slow up your productivity.

Find Your Own Spot

Where is the best place for you to put your writing talents to work? In the library? Your home? A room of your own? Whatever your choice, find a comfortable and quiet spot free of distractions. Your privacy is essential. Make sure the telephone is out of sight and sound, for once it rings and you respond, those precious thoughts may be lost forever.

Since writing is a solitary pursuit, your unavailability to family and friends at certain periods must be respected as well as understood. Although they may get a bit testy about it, just wait until your article is accepted. They will be the first to tout your success.

Choose Your Modus Operandi

With your schedule intact and your working site determined, you now must decide on the most effective way to write your article. Authors have their favorites. Rejecting the word processor, novelist Danielle Steel does all her writing on her longtime faithful typewriter. Those enamored of their computers, however, find word processing the only way to get their thoughts out as quickly as they come.

Still others who may need more time to reflect, prefer to write first in longhand. Another approach, that of speaking into a tape recorder or dictaphone, encourages the free flow of ideas. At the same time, the material must be transcribed, thus making the process time consuming and costly in some cases.

Whatever your modus operandi, don't neglect your posture or vision. Writing is best done while sitting in a straight back chair at a table or desk with adequate lighting. In preparing for the first draft, gather your tools and supplies around you. Resources such as style guides, *Roget's International Thesaurus,* *Webster's Collegiate Dictionary,* and a dictionary of synonyms and antonyms will become your indispensable companions as you begin to write.

FIRMING UP YOUR FIRST DRAFT

So far, you have successfully completed a number of steps in the writing process. As you begin to write, feel confident that you will be able to achieve a satisfactory first draft. Let the 3Rs guide you along this journey: *ramble, ramble,* and *ramble.* In no way does this imply a laissez faire technique. After all, you have an excellent outline to show you the direction.

Rambling is quite functional in that it averts blocks and causes the work to move at a fairly rapid pace. At this stage, don't worry about form, grammar, and punctuation. *Your job is to get those ideas down as highlighted in the outline.* Let them flow in sequence although you may wish to add new thoughts and build on others as they come to mind.

This early draft of your paper should be as full as possible. No need to be concerned if any of the information no longer seems relevant. It is always easier to delete unwanted material later than to fill in areas done too sketchily.

Beginning authors tend to experience two common pitfalls that make writing stressful. They take too long in getting started, and when finally underway they write too slowly and tediously. Furthermore, they pause interminably at the end of a sentence or paragraph and then go back to read and edit what they have done. This process is counterproductive and should be avoided. Otherwise, after a while the person wonders if the article will ever be finished.

Practicing the 3Rs will eliminate this problem. Make a tentative start with an introductory statement even if you decide to change it later. Write quickly without pausing for mechanics (such as hyphens, commas) or checking spellings. If you need to stop for a moment, do so between paragraphs or the larger sections of your article. Writing interrupted by pauses, however, will suffer as a result, to say nothing of your work schedule.

In this initial try, write as much of the work as you can, preferably to the end. If you have to take time out, read what has been written before picking up where you left off.

Whether you write in longhand or use a computer or typewriter, allow plenty of space on the paper with generous margins and double or triple spacing between sentences. In this way, you allow for filling gaps or citing changes after completing the first draft.

When you complete the draft, you will have overcome a gigantic hurdle. Your paper may seem like a jigsaw puzzle at this point but that will change. As you rewrite and rewrite, you will see the evolution of your article from a rough cut into a polished, professional looking work. It make take two, three, or more drafts, but you will be ready to meet that challenge.

SUMMARY

When writers begin the first draft, they have reached a milestone in the writing process. With the preliminary steps completed, the real test comes in converting what has been learned into the written word. The success of that effort will depend upon the self-discipline the person brings to the work, the nature of the topic, and the skill shown in presenting it.

LESSON 7
SELF-TEST

Circle the appropriate answer below.   **True** **False**

1. People who think clearly should be able to write clearly.   T   F

2. A sentence should be able to express more than one
   dominant thought.   T   F

3. It is acceptable to connect separate thoughts with
   conjunctions such as and or but.   T   F

4. Simple sentences used frequently make it easier to read.   T   F

5. Compound sentences should be used when you want to
   give equal emphasis to two related ideas.   T   F

6. Transition paragraphs are often used to separate or
   summarize certain areas.   T   F

7. If you're not in the mood to write, you shouldn't push it.   T   F

8. Word processing is an effective method to use because
   you can work more quickly this way.   T   F

9. Rambling through your first draft is a great deterrent
   to writer's block.   T   F

10. In most cases, revision can be completed in less than
    three drafts.   T   F

Lesson 8

How to Be Your Own Editor

You may think revision begins only with the second draft, but it really is a part of every stage of the writing process. Just think of the many times you had to revise your topic to arrive at an acceptable thesis statement. What about the reworking of your method of development or your outline?

Some of the greatest poets, scholars, and essayists began their work with ordinary thoughts in careless language, which they eventually refined through numerous revisions. So don't despair when you look at your initial rough draft and see imperfections. If you did your job of focusing on the main concepts to be incorporated, there is no basis for concern. Let style and correctness rest temporarily on the back burner while you attend to the larger elements.

Your initial task is to review the paper as a whole, reading it with a fresh, critical eye. However, give yourself a few days away from it, so you can return to the draft with a new perspective. Then, read it aloud since the ear picks up things that the eye doesn't always catch.

Ask yourself these questions: How does the paper read? How does it sound? How does it feel? Can you pinpoint something that doesn't seem quite right? The time has come for you to assess your paper with precise criteria. In other words, you will learn how to become your own editor.

You will begin this rigorous process with your second draft by testing for content followed by organization. Don't be disappointed if these two major areas require more than one or two revisions. The rewrite will depend on the extent of the work to be done. After improving your content and organization, you can then test for style and clarity of expression. Checking for spelling and punctuation will be next, along with feedback from an expert in your field to firm up your revision.

TESTING FOR CONTENT

Your first draft should ensure that enough material has been included to achieve the article's purpose. Therefore, you will need to address the following criteria.

The Article Is Substantive

The first step is to determine if your thesis statement has been developed to its fullest. Have you clearly conveyed to the reader your central message? This aim is achieved when all topic sentences build on the thesis and, in turn, are supported by concrete and relevant matter.

You also want to determine if the draft has fulfilled your original promise of providing new, timely, and significant information. Another point is to make sure that the content reflects language appropriate to the audience you wish to reach. Decide if further strengthening might be needed with the use of examples, anecdotes, and dialogue.

The Article Is Accurate and Precise

Every author must be a responsible reporter. If you falter and don't check and document properly, your credibility will be questioned. And your reputation is important to you as a person and a professional.

Be thorough as well as factual when you make statements. Examine your interpretations and generalizations to be certain they are reasonable as well as persuasive. If you quote or paraphrase authorities, be precise. Do not present information out of context or give an unbalanced view.

TESTING FOR ORGANIZATION

It is more the rule than the exception for writers to cut and paste as they revise their manuscript. Although your outline may have suggested a logical order with headings and supporting statements, some reshuffling may be indicated when you start to write.

The Introduction Draws Your Audience

Your lead will be the key to "grabbing" the reader's interest from the beginning of the article. Your title also has a role to play. If it is imaginative while defining the topic, the chances are that the editor will retain it. Otherwise, the journal will pick its own.

Your lead is extremely crucial because it introduces the main theme. If it doesn't quite have the right touch, then find a new one. Or, look further down in the paper for a lead that is just dying to be relocated! Whatever you decide on, don't waste that precious space.

The Body Sustains Your Audience

As you move into the body of the paper, does your narrative hold the reader's attention? Is your subject advanced by providing clear cut stages, and does it reveal the relationship between one stage and the next?

Your paragraphs must show continuity by making appropriate transitions. A paragraph that sounds like a new beginning, as if nothing has already been said, will require some work. The problem could be that it appears in the wrong place, or the topic sentence needs revision.

Paragraphs also reflect your point of view and method of development. Be fairly consistent when you use first, second, or third person. Avoid hopping around or you will confuse your reader.

Have you scrutinized your writing in relation to the form selected? If your approach is description, check to see if you have emphasized the right points, found the right words for them, and placed them in the best order.

Supposing your approach has been argumentation mainly, ask yourself if you are presenting your case clearly, honestly, objectively, and with good reasoning. Determine whether or not more evidence is required.

The Conclusion Satisfies Your Audience

As you come to the end of your article, does it bring your topic to a logical close? Your readers must be left with a definite feeling about the central message you want them to carry away. Avoid bringing in any irrelevant or extraneous matters or your story will go flat on you—the last thing you want to happen. If you believe that recommendations are indicated, be sure to include them. Always put the general suggestions before the specific ones.

TESTING FOR STYLE AND CLARITY OF EXPRESSION

After examining the content and organization of your draft, you will need to look at the language used and the quality of the words, sentences, and paragraphs that make up its style. You will read some passages that impress you as being clear, accurate, and direct, whereas others may seem awkward, shapeless, and lacking in movement. Your job is to identify any of these defects and to remedy them. That's what revision is all about.

Writing in a crisp, straightforward manner should be the goal of every potential author. Too often, the main idea fails to get across because it is buried in a cloud of rhetoric gushing with pedantic prose and jargon. You can avoid this serious shortcoming by heeding the following questions in relation to words and sentences.

Words

- Are all the words necessary? Too many adjectives, adverbs? Clichés? Repetition of words and phrases?

- Are you using active verbs rather than the passive voice, as well as eliminating the verb "to be" (is, was, has) as much as possible?

- Are there words that should be deleted because they add nothing to the thought?

- Do you tend to begin sentences consecutively with the word "The"? (a boring practice)

- Do you use modifiers properly?

Sentences

- Does each sentence flow naturally from the preceding one or does it seem disconnected?

- Are the sentences unwieldy or do they flow easily to the end?

- Do you have an adequate number of sentences in each paragraph?

- Do your topic sentences set the tone for the rest of the paragraph?

- Are the sentences grammatically correct? Proper use of complex sentences?

TESTING FOR THE MECHANICS

Punctuation aims to bring together some words and to separate others. It marks the pauses and emphasis for writers to use to enhance their prose. Commas, semicolons, and periods give important pauses to the printed page.

If commas seem to give you a bit of trouble, here's how to use them:

1. Before *and, but, for, or, nor, yet, still* when joining independent clauses.

2. Between all terms in a series, *including the last two.*

3. To set off parenthetical openers and afterthoughts.

4. Before and after parenthetical insertions (use a *pair* of commas).

Sometimes semicolons are overused and should be employed guardedly. They are most effective in a series of clauses or phrases.

Writers need to bone up on the various uses of punctuation such as the colon, parentheses, dash, brackets, quotation marks, italics, ellipsis, and others. One rule on hyphens remains solid: hyphenate two or more words serving together as an adjective. Also, have your dictionary in hand to know how to hyphenate properly.

When it comes to spelling, the dictionary is again your best friend. Editors cringe when they see misspellings, particularly the more common *accommodate, acknowledgment, commitment,* and *judgment.* If you have one of the word processing programs that check spellings, then use it and more power to you. Remember, however, that most of these programs will not catch a correctly spelled word in the wrong place (bat for but, for example), so a careful reading is still advised.

TEST FOR FEEDBACK

When you have done your best work in revising your article and have typed what you hope will be nearly the last draft, read your manuscript aloud. Proof the copy twice, the first time to hear how it sounds and the second time to spot any typos, misspellings, or punctuation errors. As a final check, try proofing backwards as it will allow you to see every word without jumping ahead.

Your article will be in good enough shape to share with someone in your field—a colleague, instructor, or some other authority—whose expertise, objectivity, and confidence you respect. *Feedback from one person should suffice.*

After receiving the critique, rework your paper into its final form to submit to the editor of your target journal. Your mission is almost completed!

SUMMARY

Few people can write so well that the first draft represents their best effort. Rewriting is the essence of good writing. You begin by critiquing its larger elements, your content and organization, which will make your topic interesting as well as accurate. As you perfect and polish up your style, the work will have a vitality that will take your readers on a smooth journey from beginning to end.

Meticulous attention to mechanics, careful proofreading, and some solid feedback from an expert will hasten the delivery of your article to the editor's desk.

LESSON 8
SELF-TEST

Circle the appropriate answer below.   **True   False**

1. It is more desirable to focus on content and organization than other elements in the second draft.   T   F

2. When critiquing your paper, you can automatically assume that all the information is new, timely, and significant.   T   F

3. You can feel secure adhering to your outline as you revise your paper.   T   F

4. Once you get the reader's attention with a good lead, you can feel confident in sustaining that interest.   T   F

5. It is inadvisable to add extraneous material as you conclude the article.   T   F

6. As you revise the second draft, the more content you add will enhance the substance of the piece.   T   F

7. All sentences in a paragraph should relate to the topic sentence.   T   F

8. Good punctuation helps but it is not that important.   T   F

9. Careless spelling means a careless paper.   T   F

10. It is desirable to have the opinion of more than one expert to review your paper because more input will be helpful.   T   F

Lesson 9

Behind the Editor's Desk

You can't believe it! What may have seemed a bit chaotic in your first draft has developed into an article with form and substance. Finally, the moment you have waited and worked for has arrived after constant refinement. You are ready to submit your treasured opus to the journal of choice.

PREPARING YOUR MANUSCRIPT

By now you should be thoroughly familiar with the publication's guidelines for authors, which give specific information about manuscript preparation. Although editors may have individual differences as to manuscript length, number of copies to be submitted, types of references, payment, and so on, there are basic requirements applicable to all journals. Here are some pointers to help you.

- Never send a manuscript to more than one journal at a time.

- Type manuscript double spaced on one side on white bond paper, $8^1/_2 \times 11$ inches, with minimal margins of $1^1/_4$ inches. (Legible computer printouts are acceptable in some cases.)

- Send manuscript unstapled or unclipped (unless otherwise specified) with cover letter in manila envelope. Enclose the requested number of copies.

- Send first class mail rather than certified or registered mail (except for valuable contents).

- Paginate in upper right corner flush with margin.

- Omit author's name on text if it is a refereed journal. Use title page for name and manuscript title.

- Retain at least one copy of manuscript for your files.

- Some journals request computer disks along with your manuscript. Keep this in mind if you use a word processor.

Use of Photographs and Other Visuals

Journal guidelines spell out policies regarding photographs, slides, charts, tables, and other visuals. Whereas some editors request black and white glossy photos, 5 × 7 inches or 8 × 10 inches of crisp, clear quality, others suggest color prints or slides and sometimes negatives. Be sure to secure the photographer's name for a credit line. In addition, if you submit pictures of patients or identifiable people, you will need signed releases. If you work in a hospital or university, the public relations or publicity departments can advise you on the matter.

When enclosing photos with your manuscript, protect them well against bending or tearing. Never write in ink on the back of them, or use a paper clip. Instead, type captions identifying the content on stick-on labels and affix them to the back of the photograph. Also, if you want your visuals returned (as well as your manuscript if rejected), enclose a stamped, self addressed envelope.

Citing Your References

The documentation provided in your article adds to its breadth as well as your credibility. Timely and authoritative sources must be referenced with care. Editors clearly stipulate the preferred method, with some favoring the *APA* format or *Index Medicus* or suggesting some other approach.

References should be cited on the last page and typed double spaced. They may appear alphabetically by the author's name, or in numerical order cited in the text. List only those references included in the body of your paper. A bibliography may not be required. The best way to see if you are on the right track is to check the guidelines and the journal itself.

Policy on Payment

When your article is accepted for publication, what kind of reimbursement, if any, can you expect? Unlike magazines in the commercial arena which usually pay on acceptance, most health care journals compensate in some way *after* the article appears in print. Although the monetary return may seem quite scanty after all your hard work, remember the other perks that come from publishing—*recognition in your field, growth in your career,* and *greater self-esteem.*

The journal guidelines will inform you of its policy on payment. One publication may pay $20 a page, whereas another offers an honorarium from $200 to $300 for an eight-page article. The majority of journals give "tear sheets" or reprints, or a few complimentary copies of the issue containing your article. In cases where an author would like more reprints, these can be purchased at the time of publication.

AT THE EDITORIAL HELM

Once you post your manuscript to your selected journal, it is literally out of your hands. All you can do is wait anxiously, and hope for the best. The fate of your prized work rests with someone else who will determine its future (and maybe yours).

You may wonder about these esteemed people who sit in the editorial catbird seat, wielding considerable power. In the health care press, particularly the nursing journals, their influence today travels far and wide. This is a far cry from over a century ago when the *Trained Nurse and Hospital Review* was the first and only journal of that period.

When nursing expanded its scope of practice and clinical specialists and nurse practitioners came into their own in the 1970s and 1980s, however, the deluge came. New organizations and nursing journals soon followed and are still flourishing. You can be sure that as soon as a new subspecialty emerges, a journal won't be far behind. What this means is that nursing and related journals are reaching out to a broad and diversified audience to deliver their messages.

How Editors Get There

One of the best ways to know editors is through their editorials. Some write superb opinion pieces that are pungent and provocative, and excite their readers. Just think of your favorites. Most nursing editors are women and registered nurses in the age range of 35 to 55 years. Only a small number have come up through the ranks as assistant or associate editors. Few have been trained as journalists or professional editors. All, however, are experts in the content area of the journal they edit. With the marked growth of nursing publications, a group of nurse editors met a few years ago to form the International Academy of Nursing Editors. The organization has expanded substantially and meets annually to share mutual concerns.

Prior to their present post, editors served on journal editorial or advisory boards, reviewed manuscripts, and published some articles. Many claimed to have read widely the nursing literature as well as participated in several professional organizations.

How Editors Operate

Editors of nursing journals operate in one of two ways. Several work full time at their journal offices, such as the *American Journal of Nursing, Nurse Educator, Nursing, Nursing Management,* and others. The majority, however, are part-time editors who hold regular positions in clinical practice, education, administration, or consultation. For example, Peggy Chinn, editor of *Advances in Nursing Science,* and Donna Diers, editor of *Image, Journal of Nursing Scholarship,* both have academic appointments.

What Editors Do

Whether full time or part time, all editors screen manuscripts that reach their desk. If the article seems to have merit, it may be shared with the editorial staff (if in house) or sent directly to referees for review. When a manuscript does not seem suitable, it will be rejected and the author notified.

The editor establishes the journal's operational policies, as well as the editorial policies, sometimes in consort with an editorial board and/or staff. If the publication is the official organ of a professional association, such as the *AORN Journal* or the *Journal of Professional Nursing,* its editorials will reflect the positions of that organization.

Below are some of the other activities of editors:

- Recruit and work with reviewers and editorial advisors.

- Correspond and work with authors.

- Solicit manuscripts of quality.

- Perform some substantive editing.

Editors find their jobs intellectually stimulating. The challenge comes from spotting new talent, a "discovery" perhaps, and determining appropriate manuscripts. There is the joy of helping to contribute to the body of knowledge as well as being in a key position in the profession. When you're the editor, everybody wants you! But always remember that editors need you as much as you need them.

PROCESSING YOUR MANUSCRIPT

An editor's initial impression of a manuscript can make all the difference as to whether or not it will be pursued further. If it is typed clearly and neatly, accompanied by a succinct, well-written cover letter, you have already scored some brownie points. When a topic looks interesting, an editor may be motivated to read through the entire manuscript as quickly as possible.

In most situations, however, such an expectation may be unrealistic. When the journal approaches its production deadline or the editor is away at a conference or ready to go out of town, priorities can change.

"How long then should I wait for a reply?" you ask. Even though there may be no decision as yet on the disposition of your paper, you usually can count on some acknowledgment within a month after submitting it. Editors or their assistants often send a post card or letter to the author indicating that the work has been received and is being considered by the journal's staff, or referred to outside experts for critique. Although a review does not imply a near acceptance, it signifies that the manuscript has passed the editor's screening.

If you do not hear from the journal in a month's time, don't hesitate to write to the editor. You never know when a manuscript gets lost in the mail or is misrouted or misplaced among the mass of paper circulating around a magazine's offices. You could write a simple, cordial letter as follows:

February 11, 1992

Maribel S. Stewart, MS, RN
Editor
Health Horizons
5 Hyde Park
Park Ridge, IL 60698

Dear Ms. Stewart:

I wonder if any conclusion has been reached about my manuscript, "Millie Smith: Public Health Rebel," that I sent to you on January 8, 1992.

Your attention to this matter will be greatly appreciated.

Sincerely yours,

Clara Lou Stokes, MA, RN

More than likely your letter will be acknowledged in a short time. If you don't hear within two or three weeks, by all means telephone the editor. You have a right to know if your manuscript has been received.

THE REFEREED JOURNAL—WHAT IT MEANS

Some people view the concept of a refereed journal as a fairly new phenomenon. On the contrary, however, its roots go back to the mid-18th century when the Royal Society of England introduced the idea to improve the quality of articles appearing in *Philosophical Transaction,* the first medical journal. Decades later, many editors still believe that the objective and expert guidance of peer reviewers helps to maintain higher standards of professional publications.

As health care journals continue to proliferate, many have followed the trend of peer review. Glance over some of these journals (generally the second or third page) and you will see the names of authorities listed as members of editorial or advisory boards, panels, or committees. In most cases, such individuals serve as referees or reviewers of manuscripts that relate to their own area of expertise. They are known for their publications and other professional contributions.

As your name begins to get into print, you too may qualify as a reviewer in time. All journal editors maintain a roster of several names to handle this work. There are usually three or more reviewers who judge the merit of each manuscript based on criteria set by the journal. More than half of the articles undergo what is called blind review, in which the author is anonymous. Only the editor knows the person's identity. The other method of peer review is when the name appears on the manuscript.

Whether or not the author is known, the refereeing process should be completed within eight weeks after receiving the article. Although the format of the criteria varies among journals, certain areas are highlighted, such as general qualities (comprehensiveness, conciseness), value or significance, originality, reliability, and clarity of writing style. In addition to these criteria, reviewers are expected to make constructive comments on their manuscript copies, which are returned to the journal editor with a letter summarizing their remarks. Each referee has three options concerning the manuscript's potential: (1) *accept without revisions,* (2) *accept with revisions,* and (3) *do not accept.*

When reviews are forwarded to the journal, the editor transfers the comments and questions to a copy of the manuscript, which is sent to the author for revision. In some instances, certain sections of a reviewer's copy may be duplicated or incorporated into the editor's letter.

A response suggesting revision should be viewed as quite positive. Although it cannot be construed as a firm commitment to publish, it is an encouraging sign. As the author in such a situation, you would want to accept the challenge and start revising immediately. Also, inform the editor of your decision and indicate when you plan to complete the revision if a deadline has not already been given to you.

If your manuscript has been accepted without any revision, you are indeed a rare bird! And you deserve to gloat. But what about the person whose hopes of publishing have been dampened temporarily by a letter of rejection? Yes, it is disappointing, but it may console you to know that all authors, even the seasoned pros who have published extensively, admit to having a manuscript or two rejected at one time or another in their career. What you need to do is review the reasons for the rejection. If you still believe in your article, try another journal.

What are the benefits as well as some of the imperfections of the refereeing process? The chief advantage of vigorous peer review is that it should foster the publishing of articles of quality and weed out the undesirable ones. Its strength lies in the qualifications and conscientiousness of the reviewers and journal editors. If you are a health professional working in a college or university, you know all about the ongoing push to publish. Promotion, tenure, and research funding greatly depend on your record in peer review journals.

Two important points must be stressed in regard to the external review of manuscripts. On the down side, a commonly expressed concern is the objectivity of the reviewer. In most situations the risk is minimal, but there have been instances of the person's bias interfering with a just critique. A referee, for example, who does not share the same values, perspective, or non-traditional ideas espoused in a particular manuscript may reject it solely on that basis even though the work is sound and acceptable. Fortunately, other reviewers also evaluate the same article.

In the final analysis, however, editors of journals make the decision whether or not to publish after considering all the reviews. Their wisdom and editorial judgment will determine the quality and fairness of the critiques and the acceptability of the manuscript.

Another point to be made is that a journal without referees does not necessarily publish inferior material. Some of these publications are headed by first rate editors who offer articles of exceedingly high quality. In the long run, it will be the reader who determines the excellence of articles and the worthiness of the journals in which they appear—whether refereed or not.

ACCEPTANCE AND THE NEXT STEPS

What happens to your manuscript after it has been accepted? Here is an example of how a letter from an editor (or senior editor) may inform an author of the good news:

Dear Ms. Stokes:

After carefully reviewing your manuscript, "Millie Smith: Public Health Rebel," we are happy to inform you that we believe it will make a contribution to Health Horizons. *The article will be scheduled for an upcoming issue. . . .*

The letter may also indicate the length of the editing process, which can run from eight to twelve months in some cases. It will mention remuneration and probably request some biographical data as well as a signed statement transferring copyright to the journal. The copyright form means that if an individual, in the future, wants to duplicate your article or extensively quote from it, permission must be obtained from you *and* the journal.

It is important for all writers to be aware of copyright requirements, including the use of visuals from other sources. If you want to copy or adapt a diagram or some other artwork, you must get approval in writing. Conversely, any individual who wishes to use an original design or model appearing in your article, will need to get your permission to reproduce it. Lesson 10 details more fully other copyright practices.

Editing Your Manuscript

If you have not heard further about your manuscript in six months after acceptance, call or write to the editor to ascertain its status. The edited version may even be on its way to you.

Every journal reserves the right to edit all manuscripts according to its style and space requirements and to clarify content. Copy editors, managing editors, and other staff may all have a hand in the process.

A copy editor works mainly on stylistic details or changes, using the editing style or guidelines adopted by the journal. It is not unusual for the top editor to put a blue pencil to the copy, concentrating on the accuracy, substance, and flow of the content.

If your article has followed the principles of good writing and you have studied the style of the articles appearing in your target journal, your manuscript should not require heavy editing. When authors complain about the marked changes made on their manuscripts, it is usually because they have been lax in the above two areas. Be grateful that there are editorial experts to put that finishing touch to your paper. Their credo is: "We take a good thing and make it better!"

After your manuscript has been edited, the journal will send you the copy for approval. Usually, the article has been set in type as it will appear in the issue. You may receive a set of galleys (vertical column strips) or page proofs. Your job is *not* to rewrite copy or change words, but rather to look at any content alterations or distortions from the original copy. You may find certain sentences or paragraphs deleted for space reasons. If these omissions affect the continuity or integrity of the article, you must inform the editor. You don't want to mislead your readers. Otherwise, don't get too "picky" since changes can be costly.

Scheduling Your Article

When the copy is approved by the author, the journal issue carrying your article may already be scheduled for production. Unlike newspapers which have short deadlines, the cutoff dates for journals, particularly a monthly journal, is from two to three months in advance of publication. Space is only held for last-minute news stories. Although your article may be set for a certain issue, don't be too disappointed if it is postponed. Other priorities can delay your story, but it will be printed eventually. Contact the editor about rescheduling if you haven't been informed.

The time period from the acceptance of a manuscript to publication varies from journal to journal. The decision is contingent upon the backlog of accepted manuscripts, scheduling changes, the publication's frequency (monthly, bimonthly, quarterly), and other factors.

REWARDS OF AUTHORSHIP

Once you know when your article comes off the press, you will count the days until the journal comes in the mail. Whether you have published once, twice, or many times, it is always a thrill to see your work, your very own creation, come to life in the pages of a major health care journal.

Perhaps more than one complimentary copy will reach you at the same time. As mentioned earlier, some of the rewards include reprints, tear sheets, or an honorarium. If you coauthored a paper, then you and your colleague will share the bounty (if a check, it will usually be made out to just one author).

Becoming a published writer is not only a great enhancement of self-esteem; it also makes the institution where you work look good. If you are connected with a university, hospital, or other health care facility, show copies of your article to the public relations/publicity people. If they find it significant, they might issue a news release to the health press. Also, if there is an in-house newsletter or magazine, let the editor know about your story.

You have worked hard in the process of becoming an author. After a period of gestation, you gave birth to a wonderful idea, nurtured it, and saw it grow. Each stage generated new learning until your idea developed into an entity of substance and worth.

You are already thinking about your next article. The effort will require a lot of self-discipline, but the steps will come easier. You have made the long day's journey into successful authorship. Congratulations and continuing success!

SUMMARY

The final stage of the writing process is like pulling together all the loose ends and wrapping them up in a neat little package. After arduous revision, your manuscript is in its best form and ready to go. You will enter the editorial world and learn something about the mystique behind the editor's desk, all the way from the refereeing process to acceptance and publishing of your article.

You have done your lessons in a systematic fashion, and the proof of your efforts is in the product. Although interesting, the process has not been easy, but whatever the obstacles and detours you have overcome them. It is a journey that you can expect to travel many times.

LESSON 9
SELF-TEST

Circle the appropriate answer below.   **True False**

1. A manuscript can be sent to more than one editor at a
time as long as you inform the editor.   T   F

2. A journal automatically returns a rejected manuscript
to the author.   T   F

3. Only cite references at the end of an article that have
been included in the text.   T   F

4. Most health care journals give honoraria to authors.   T   F

5. If a journal is refereed, the reviewer does not know the
identity of the author.   T   F

6. A copy editor deals with stylistic changes in most cases. T   F

7. The refereed process has more positives than negatives.   T   F

8. The editor generally has the final say on the disposition
of manuscripts.   T   F

9. Most nursing journal editors worked on the editorial
staff prior to their present post.   T   F

10. Authors with accepted manuscripts should not bother
editors about the status of their manuscripts regarding
scheduling.   T   F

Lesson 10

Ethics in Journalism: What Health Professionals Need to Know

*I*s ethics in the health care field an endangered species when it relates to responsible journalism? The question should evoke considerable interest since health professionals publish increasingly and new journals continue to thrive.

The attention given to ethical behavior in the health disciplines is nothing new—it has been instilled in practitioners from day one. With the advent of technology, however, as well as complex protocols and procedures, nurses, physicians, researchers, and others find themselves dealing more and more with ethical matters. Just look at the compendium of literature and the numerous seminars, conferences, and workshops on the topic.

Ethics appears to be "in," at least in the patient care setting. But isn't it ironic that this important value seems to be losing out in the realm of scholarly and journalistic communication? What can account for the flagrant violation of ethical principles that is on the rise in health care journals?

Lest it seem unfair to single out the health care community, the problem should be examined within the context of the larger society and what appears to be its changing value system. Grinspan (1988) points out how the country has inherited a legacy of a quarter century of social disruptions. On the coattails of the Vietnam War, Watergate, the assassinations of John Fitzgerald Kennedy and Martin Luther King, and other tragedies have come the more recent scandals in the world of Wall Street, athletics, government, and international politics.

The climate of distrust is pervasive. American consumers don't know what to believe or not to believe. Although many members of the media, print and otherwise, continue to report responsibly, they seem to be overshadowed by the growth of sleazy tabloids and scurrilous talk show programs that prey upon the most intimate aspects of people's lives. Of course, if it's not your thing, don't read, watch, or listen to such media!

That kind of a response may be peremptory, particularly when there are substantive ways of dealing with the more fundamental ethical and moral issues of contemporary life. A good beginning to recoup some of our lost faith in human values might be in raising them to full consciousness and studying them critically.

Even with the abuses evident in the communication arena, the overriding benefit of a democratic nation is the right to free speech enunciated in the First Amendment, the foundation of our ethical system. As Jefferson rightly pointed out, when the press is free and every man able to read, all is safe.

Journalists, like other professionals, have codes to guide them in the conduct of their work. As Mencher (1987, p. 617) notes, however, no code can make a person of good conscience. "Only a personal commitment to a journalistic morality can determine that."

The concept of a code of ethics in the nursing profession can be traced to 1893 when Lystra Gretter wrote the Florence Nightingale pledge, designed to guide ethical behavior (Kalisch & Kalisch, 1988). Isabel Hampton Robb (1990, p. 16) reinforced this idea at the turn of the century when she defined ethics as "the rule of conduct adapted to the many diverse circumstances attending nursing of the sick." Twenty-six years later, the first suggested code of ethics was presented to the delegates of the American Nurses Association at their convention (A Code of Ethics, 1926).

Through the years, nursing's code of ethics has undergone changes, refinement, and interpretation. It aims to guide nurses in *all* aspects of professional life. Implicit in that intent is a commitment to follow ethical principles in every professional endeavor. Surely, within that context, professional and scholarly writing should loom high as an important responsibility.

In the journalism field, Sigma Delta Chi, as the professional society, enunciates a code of ethics applicable to writers in any discipline. The code emphasizes that journalists carry obligations requiring them to perform with intelligence, objectivity, accuracy, and fairness (Meyer, 1987).

PRACTICING THE BASIC VALUES

Accuracy was the cardinal rule for the staff of Joseph Pulitzer, yesterday's giant of American journalism. You may also remember the wonderful stories of *The New Yorker's* A.J. Liebling, who paid the highest compliment to his colleagues when he characterized them as careful reporters.

Accuracy means getting the facts straight. If you quote directly from an authority, do it correctly and within the appropriate context. Be accurate even when you paraphrase the remarks of another person. A good precept to follow is: *Do unto others as you wish them to do unto you.* Be meticulous about names, dates, page numbers, and whatever else is needed.

Fairness and objectivity are other values for every writer to follow. Your story requires balance and straightforwardness, which means freedom from bias. *Depend on the evidence, not on opinion.* An article must also be complete since no work is fair if it provides half truths or omits information of major importance. Furthermore, if you add irrelevant material at the expense of significant facts, you mislead your audience with a distorted and dishonest view of the real picture.

Fair play implies being up front with authorities whom you contact for interviews. If you plan to use a tape recorder on the telephone, always obtain permission from the other party. Although it is legal in most states to tape record without informing the interviewee, this practice cannot be condoned. It is far better for the individual to know that the conversation is for the record. Like many responsible newspapers, the *Washington Post* does not permit its reporters to tape calls unless the other person agrees (Meyer, 1987).

Protecting Your Copyright

Why should authors be concerned with copyright vis-à-vis ethical questions? Because it is a form of protection provided by the laws of the United States (title 17, U.S. Code), to prevent others from copying your work (U.S. Copyright Office, 1988). Ever since 1790, Article I, Section 8 has given Congress the power to secure for authors and inventors the exclusive right to their writings and discoveries. Only two major revisions in the copyright law have occurred during the 20th century—in 1909 and 1976.

The newer revision covers works created after January 1, 1978, for a term lasting the author's lifetime and 50 years after death. Works protected under the old law are covered for 75 years.

When you write for a journal or publishing house, the editor sends you a form to fill out transferring copyright ownership. Some authors negotiate for first rights, and if agreeable to the publisher they retain the copyright. This practice, however, rarely occurs with health care publications.

The absence of copyright protection does not mean that new authorship would cease, but unauthorized reproduction and distribution would stifle the quantity and diversity of creative activity. Quality, of course, would take a back seat.

Copyright infringement consists of violating any of the exclusive rights of a copyright owner, such as making an unauthorized copy of a work. It does not involve copying the "ideas" (See next section on plagiarism), but is concerned that the manner of expressing them not be reproduced.

Unless a publication specifies otherwise, the general rule is that a person who wishes to extract material from a published source may generally do so up to 500 words from a book (of about 500 pages), or approximately 200 words from a 2,000-word article. In most cases, permission is not required but proper attribution must be given. If you look inside the cover of a book or journal, you will see the copyright symbol and the year. For example: *Copyright © 1992 National League for Nursing Press. All rights reserved.*

For many years, academics were regarded as the greatest offenders of the copyright law, with their indiscriminate photocopying of books, articles, pictorial and graphic work, and other copyrighted material. This practice underwent reform after the 1976 revision with its stringent requirements and enforcement by the U.S. Copyright Office. In December 1982, the Association of American Publishers (AAP) brought a successful suit for the first time for copyright infringement against a major private university.

The AAP charged the university, several faculty members, and a nearby copy center with asking students to buy copies of published materials. There had been no request for permission, or any payment of royalties by any of the charged parties. Such unlawful practices tend to deprive authors and publishers of their rightful fees.

Most libraries in colleges and universities issue guidelines for students and faculty about copyrighted works. Many photocopy businesses, particularly those located near academic institutions, have become fair targets for inspectors checking compliance with the copyright law. In some cases, costly law suits have been filed against these establishments.

The issue of copyrighting has assumed a new dimension with the impact of information technologies on scholarly methods and publishing. With new concerns raised about nonprint formats, such as videotapes and consumer software, the potential for copyright infringement has increased. If you are a faculty member or a graduate student, you should be particularly aware of your school's policies on copyrighted materials.

Lamenting Literary Theft

Are copyright infringement and plagiarism two sides of the same coin? Quite possibly yes, but there are distinct differences although people tend to confuse them.

Plagiarism, otherwise known as literary theft, is the passing off of another person's ideas or writings as your own, without giving credit to the source. To put it more bluntly, plagiarism is stealing or what Zorn (1981, p. 1) characterizes as "brazen shoplifting in the marketplace of words and ideas." Unhappily, the record is long and universal, filled with names of the most illustrious writers in history from Dickens and Chaucer to some well known contemporary folks. But that doesn't make it right. It's not so funny if you are the one being plagiarized.

Discussing famous authors who have cribbed from earlier writers, Zorn (1981, p. 2) points out that "even with such a noble legacy, writers who steal from others are held in the greatest contempt by fellow scribes."

Some people even become boastful of their thievery, almost believing that the lifted ideas could be their own. Leo (1988) comments on one offender who acknowledged that he knew what he was doing, which was acting as a populizer making history come alive!

Critical of the publish-or-perish system which Leo (1988) says encourages quantity and not quality, he chastises the academic community:

> *The byproducts of this curious system are not only unreadable articles but also the rise of thousands of academic journals that are not actually meant to be read. . . . Besides assuring the triumph of the mediocre, the system makes plagiarism more likely. (p. 90)*

Whether intentional or not, plagiarism in academic life entails severe penalties which may involve a failing course grade to a student or even expulsion, or a sharp reprimand or suspension to a guilty faculty member. In the business world, plagiarism frequently results in law suits or some other legal action.

Several years ago a famous case involving plagiarism occurred when an astute graduate student discovered several examples of stolen material reproduced as original writing in the works of a prominent Harvard Medical School professor. The revelation stunned the academic and medical world in light of the professor's track record as an outstanding clinician, administrator, and organizational official. When interviewed, the student stated: "I had been trained. . . to check references carefully, and consult primary sources whenever possible." (Arlen, 1988, p. 31)

Zorn (1981) claims that experts in literature and psychology identify three types of plagiarists. First, there is the person who wants to imitate the work of someone that person admires but cannot perform him or herself. Second, there is the "compulsive plagiarist who becomes possessed by the words and ideas of others and becomes psychologically incapable of distinguishing his [or her] thoughts" (p. 2) from them. Third, there is the individual who copies for the purpose of making money.

With the high value placed on refereed journals as exemplars of quality and high standards, you may wonder why reviewers allow all this purloined prose to slip by. After all, referees are supposed to be knowledgeable in their own areas of expertise. Journals, as well as book publishers, need to be more judicious in the selection of these authorities, while reviewers themselves should sharpen up their critical skills. In most instances, the aggrieved author is the one who discovers the stolen material.

What recourse do writers have when plagiarism has occurred? First, be absolutely sure of your facts. Determine to what extent someone has lifted content from your opus. A sentence or two? A paragraph? Or several passages? Are the ideas copied verbatim or paraphrased? Is credit given anywhere to the original author? The realization that someone has plagiarized you is devastating. But thievery is thievery, and you must act!

Once you have the necessary data, inform the editor of the journal or publishing company which carried your article or book. You may also wish to confer with your attorney for direction, although publishers are well equipped with legal advisors to handle matters of this sort. The general rule is *not* to contact the person who has copied your work, at least at the outset of the discovery.

You should put the facts in writing for the editor (with a copy for yourself) even though you probably will telephone first. How the situation is then pursued will depend on the policies of the publisher.

In one case of blatant plagiarism that happened not too long ago, a professor of nursing at a large midwestern university came across a journal article that contained paragraphs of material copied from her own article published in another journal about two-and-a-half years earlier. The plagiarized piece even had the same title, which is what caught the professor's eye!

She immediately called the primary journal, provided the necessary information to the editor who, in turn, contacted the editor of the second journal which printed the fraudulent article. Both editors decided that a retraction in an upcoming issue would settle the matter. When the explanation appeared many months later, it was watered down and buried in an innocuous corner of the magazine. The copy merely stated that in certain parts of the article the author inadvertently neglected to give credit to the professor. Although the plagiarizer, an instructor in a baccalaureate program, was sharply reprimanded, her future chances of publishing in the nursing press are questionable. As a professional group, editors share common concerns.

This unfortunate saga, however, has another wrinkle to it. When the professor's dean learned of the incident, she decided to contact the chairperson of the nursing department at the college where the instructor worked. When confronted, the contrite young woman tearfully promised "never to do such a thing again." After the semester, she left the college and moved to another state.

This sad but true story again illustrates the consequences of the publish-or-perish phenomenon. At the same time, there is no excuse for dishonesty or plagiarizing the work of people who have *earned* their recognition.

AUTHOR ACCOUNTABILITY

According to Blancett (May, 1991a, p. 35), unethical behavior will occur until the nursing profession has "an improved system that supports colleagueship and cooperation rather than competitiveness." Yet, competition, in itself, can be an extremely healthy motivator when it encourages creativity and stimulates original thought. But when the competitor loses sight of the end, and concentrates only on the means, however questionable, the value of the outcome is dubious.

Authors compelled to publish for reasons other than a sheer love of writing or the desire to make a contribution may resort to any method to reach their goal. In addition to plagiarism, some choose the route of multiple authorship (getting his or her name in there somehow), whereas others attempt to stretch the one-story idea into 57 varieties. The road to fraud is paved with well measured intentions.

Will the Real Author Stand Up?

Ethical decisions enter into the publishing field when multiple authors of the same work are involved. Sometimes it is a little hard to believe, and even a bit preposterous, to see four, five, or more authors contributing to one piece of work under 3,500 words! With the potential for divergent writing styles of each participant, you may further wonder how an article or research report could be put together in a coherent, uniform fashion. The chances are that the task was left to the chief author or a professional editor to smooth out the rough spots.

Can a person who has contributed one or two paragraphs or a brief section to an article with other writers legitimately claim authorship? The answer is ambiguous: yes, because the individual has written something; no, because the reader is deceived into believing that the person may have contributed more than what really occurred.

The problem here is that you never know who has written what and how much. Also, people who continue to contribute mainly in a format with more than one coauthor tend to pad their curriculum vitae to the hilt. If it is promotion or tenure such individuals seek, then committees making these determinations need to study more carefully the publications of candidates, whether they appear in a refereed journal or not.

If multiple authorship encourages neophyte writers to publish eventually on their own, some benefit might be noted. In reality, however, it does not strengthen scholarship. After all, how much original writing can be done by four or more contributors on one article of modest length? Savvy editors of journals know that responsible publishing means developing your own concept, pursuing the work needed, and writing up the effort yourself or with a coauthor or coinvestigator.

In situations with more than one contributor, who should be the senior person listed on the byline? Ethically, it would seem that the individual who does most of the writing should be the first author. It is not unusual, however, to find someone listed as the senior writer because of his or her stature in the field or in the academic hierarchy. If it is a study, he or she could be the principal investigator. Even so, participation in the project as well as in the writing of the final report or article might be limited.

In another situation, where a nurse and physician have collaborated on some research, the latter may insist upon senior authorship even though the nurse writes the entire article. Who should be listed as the first author, and does it matter whether the publication is a medical or nursing journal? You may be familiar with these examples which have no easy answers and have to be worked out by the parties involved.

In her editorial, "Who Is Entitled to Authorship?" Blancett (1991b) cites the 1988 statement of the International Committee of Medical Journal Editors, which attributes authorship credit to the following, based on substantial contributions to:

1. Conception and design or analysis and interpretation of data.

2. Drafting the article or revising it critically for important intellectual content.

3. Final approval of the version to be published.

The statement stresses that all three conditions must be met.

Since only people involved in the writing of an article should rightfully be listed as coauthors, other participants such as data collectors and research assistants may be acknowledged elsewhere in the report—in a footnote at the bottom of the first page, or at the end. It would be improper to include them in the byline.

Similar principles apply to two authors as to multiple authors. For example, the first author listed is usually the more experienced writer as well as the person who has initiated the idea and has done the most work. When there is equal division of work and writing, no one can fault you for an alphabetical listing.

A partnership of this type can be quite advantageous when authors are compatible and determine arrangements for division of responsibility, scheduling, and agreement about funds (if there is payment). As with multiple authors, ground rules must be established from the outset or the effort to coauthor can become frustrating and non-productive.

How Much Is Too Much?

Just as multiple authorship has its limitations, the practice of duplicate publication raises several ethical questions. In trying to spread the literary wealth based on a solitary concept or central message, authors may be hoisted on their own petard. Could anything be more unflattering than the response of a reader who sighs: "It's the same old tune. What else is new!"

Editors are becoming increasingly aware of writers who take what was once a good idea, camouflage it with novel words and phrases tailored to different audiences, and then pass it off as new material. You can detect duplication in any one of the following five forms:

1. Same content.

2. Similar articles with minor changes.

3. Several articles where one would suffice.

4. Sequential article about a developing article.

5. Similar articles geared to different audiences (Blancett, 1991a, b)

Vessey and Gennaro (1990) cite some of the abuses that occur in research articles concerning the duplication of data. They point to least publishable units (LPUs) that involve data presented in such a way as to "create numerous manuscripts regardless of their scientific merit" (p. 67). The availability of personal computers, they state, makes it easier to prepare similar manuscripts from the data produced.

Attempts to publish reports containing superficial material show a complete lack of professional accountability. On the other hand, there are legitimate reasons for publishing more than one article from a piece of research. Vessey and Gennaro (1990, p. 67) applaud such efforts when "diverse analyses of data bases provide rich and scientific conclusions."

Regarding the non-research article, there also are circumstances in which previously published material can be reproduced, to some extent, in another journal by the same author. In this light, writers can feel comfortable if the new article focuses on a different theme or main point from the earlier work. Another example of valid duplication is when one journal wants to reproduce an article or essay appearing in another publication. In such cases, permission must be obtained from the primary journal and credit given when the work is reprinted. Also, the second journal is expected to maintain the integrity of the article and not publish it out of context.

A serious problem in the journalism field is when an author submits the same manuscript at the same time to more than one journal. In book publishing, where policies differ, it is acceptable to send proposals and manuscripts simultaneously to several publishers. When a manuscript reaches a journal, however, the editor assumes that it has not been submitted elsewhere. It wasn't too long ago that two nursing journals carried an identical article in the same month. Does the incident reflect stupidity or greed on the part of the author? Surely, the individual must have received edited copies to approve prior to publication.

EDITORIAL ACCOUNTABILITY

There is a special relationship between an editor and an author. Nothing gives an editor more pleasure than discovering a gifted new writer and helping that individual grow in the publishing world. When their association is mutually rewarding, it evolves into a successful partnership with the reader as the chief beneficiary.

Acceptance and Then What?

The above may reflect the ideal, but it does happen more often than you think. Yet editors of health care journals, like other professionals, run the gamut from great to good to so-so. Some are more experienced in the editorial process and work well with their authors. Others, particularly neophytes to publishing, are less sophisticated and don't always know how to deal with the more sensitive issues that arise. The following illustrates a situation in which the culpability was on the part of the editor and the author unwittingly became the victim.

> *A clinician in one of the health disciplines was invited by the editor of a monthly journal to write an article on a particular topic for the upcoming May issue four months hence. The editor indicated the deadline as well as the honorarium of $300 to be paid on publication. The clinician gave high priority to the assignment and submitted the manuscript in time and it was well received. She subsequently approved the galleys set in type.*
>
> *When the May issue did not contain the article, the author contacted the editor and was informed that the piece was bumped temporarily because of space needs. After waiting patiently for several months without further word, she called the journal in October, only to be told that a new editor had been appointed and would communicate with her soon.*
>
> *A month later, she received the original manuscript and a letter stating that the article was no longer suitable due to changing needs. "Feel free to send your manuscript to another journal" were the editor's concluding words.*

Although unforeseen or unusual events occur in which a journal cannot publish an accepted article (whether solicited or not), it is customary for an editor to offer the author what is known as a "kill fee" in cases where an honorarium has been promised. Although the amount represents just a part of the original fee, the gesture shows good faith on the part of the journal.

Since the clinician-author in the above incident was not familiar with the kill-fee policy, she did not question the journal. The editor, however, should have known better, and in this respect her behavior could be considered unethical. Furthermore, her comment to send the manuscript elsewhere was a bit insensitive since it had been targeted to a special audience and would require a complete rewrite for another publication.

In a comparable situation with some other journal in which an article was accepted and then withdrawn, what might an author expect if no honorarium was indicated initially? The response would have to depend on the publication's policy in such matters. The editor might wish to make amends, perhaps by providing an annual subscription, or there could be no redress at all. When the circumstances are such that a journal is going out of business, a responsible editor tries to place manuscripts already accepted with editors of other appropriate journals. In most cases, once a manuscript is accepted, it will eventually see the printed page. When journals experience a turnover in the top command, the majority of new editors honor the commitments of their predecessors.

The Editor's Editing—Too Much, Too Little?

Sometime authors believe an injustice has been done when they see the edited version of their manuscript. How much freedom should an editor have in reworking an article? Are there ethical issues to be considered?

Most writers whose work requires a modicum of polishing can appreciate the effort that goes into improving a potentially good manuscript. As emphasized in Lesson 9, a person who follows the guidelines of a particular journal and studies the style of writing in the articles, should not expect heavy editing. Editors are thrilled to receive a work that flows beautifully and presents a clear, concise picture of its message. Such papers produce almost tears of joy because so many must be rejected due to poor writing skills.

When some editing is required, the job is done with great care. Even when a few sentences must be deleted or shortened because of space requirements, an attempt is made to maintain the continuity of thought. If authors find distortions or inconsistencies of any kind in the edited copy, they must share their concerns with the journal. Editors are grateful for this feedback since they want to publish accurate material. There could be times, however, when an author simply disapproves of the corrected version because "it just doesn't read as well as my original manuscript." But in the editor's judgment, the revised copy is the more acceptable one and requires no further changes.

If you were the author in this situation, what would you do? Accept the editor's decision and count on a published article even if it isn't quite what you expected? Or should you request that the piece be withdrawn and the original manuscript returned to you? Perhaps you would prefer to submit it to another journal even though the reaction could be similar. How you decide in these matters is important to your future in publishing. The article is your creation and you feel very protective of it. You want to maintain its integrity which you believe has been impugned to some extent. You may or may not be correct.

Here is another option for you. Before firming up your decision with the journal, why not confer with an objective colleague or expert in the field, and ask for comments on the two versions, the original and the edited one. An informed response should clarify the issue and give you a fresh perspective on the entire matter.

SUMMARY

The obligation of accountability involves a shared responsibility between editors and authors. Codes of ethical behaviors have been established to guide them in the conduct of their work. The more powerful code, however, is unwritten and deeply embedded in the consciences of people.

With the rise of fraudulent practices in scholarly and journalistic efforts, stringent enforcement must be intensified. Editors of refereed journals can begin by evaluating more carefully the critiques of their reviewers. Scrupulous monitoring of copyright infringements, literary theft, multiple authorship, and duplicate publishing will help to cut down many of these common abuses.

Also culpable are institutional committees and funding agencies that make judgments on promotion, tenure, and research money. The individuals that sit on these important bodies must be accountable, and look with greater circumspection at the published works of candidates. Perhaps the larger and more urgent problem is for academics and others to deal realistically with that old chestnut of "publish-or-perish." Isn't it time to set right a disturbed value system that seems to emphasize quantity rather than quality?

This point is best summed up by Downs (1990, p. 131) in a telling commentary to the nursing community that is applicable to all health professionals:

We owe the profession the best and most valid information we can provide. To offer less is to undermine the very purpose that publication is supposed to serve. Ultimately, that purpose is tied to better care for the people for whom we care.

REFERENCES

Arlen, M. (1988, December 7). Much ado over a plagiarist. *New York Times*, 31.

Blancett, S.S. (1991a). The ethics of writing and publishing. *Journal of Nursing Administration, 21*(5), 31–36.

Blancett, S.S. (1991b). Who is entitled to authorship? *Nurse Educator, 16*(5), 3.

Downs, F.S. (1990). Editorial. Accuracy counts too. *Nursing Research, 39*(3), 131.

Grinspan, M.C. (1988). Editor. *Ethics: Another endangered species?* Memphis, TN: Rhodes College.

Kalisch, P., & Kalisch, B. (1988). *The advance of American nursing.* Boston: Little, Brown.

Leo, J. (1988, December 12). The crimson copycat. *U.S. News and World Report,* 90.

Mencher, M. (1987). *News reporting and writing.* Fourth edition. Dubuque, IA: William C. Brown.

Meyer, P. (1987). *Ethical journalism.* New York: Longman.

Robb, I.H. (1900). *Nursing ethics for hospital and private use.* Cleveland, OH: Koeckert.

Staff (1926). A suggested code. *American Journal of Nursing, 26*(9), 599–601.

U.S. Copyright Office (1988). Circular 1: *Copyright basics.* (Publication No. 202-135/60,046). Washington, DC: U.S. Printing Office.

Vessey, J.A., & Gennaro, S. (1990). Editorial. Publish and perish. *Nursing Research,* 30 (2), 67.

Zorn, E. (1981, January 22). Plagiarism. Section 2, *Chicago Tribune,* 1, 2.

Selected Bibliography on Professional Writing

American Psychological Association (3rd ed.). (1984). *Publication manual of the American Psychological Association.* Washington, DC: Author.

Associated Press (1987). *Associated Press stylebook and libel manual: The journalist's bible.* Menlo Park, CA: Addison-Wesley.

Axelrod, R.B., & Cooper, C.R. (1985). *The St. Martin's guide to writing.* New York: St. Martin's.

Bernstein, T.M. (1971). *Miss Thistlebottom's hobgoblins.* New York: Farrar, Strauss & Giroux.

Bernstein, T.M. (1975). *The careful writer.* New York: Atheneum.

Blancett, S.S. (1988). The process and politics of writing for publication. *Clinical Nurse Specialist, 1* (3), 113–117.

Chapman, R.L. (5th ed.). (1992). *Roget's international thesaurus.* New York: Harper Collins.

*Dillard, Anne (1990). *The writing life.* New York: Harper Collins.

Downs, F.S. (1985). Congratulations! You're the worst! A terrible opening sentence for a research report. *Nursing Research, 34*(2), 70.

Downs, F.S. (1985). Unidentified acceptable manuscripts. *Nursing Research, 34*(4), 197.

*Gehle, Q., & Rollo, D. (1987). *Writing essays: A process approach.* New York: St. Martin's.

*Gordon, K.E. (1984). *The transitive vampire.* New York: Times Books.

Lambuth, D. (1976). *The golden book on writing.* New York: Viking Penguin.

Lewis, J. (1982). *The New York Times manual of style and usage.* New York: Random House.

Packer, N.H., & Timpane, J. (1989). *Writing worth reading.* New York: St. Martin's.

Scholes, R., & Comley, N.R. (1989). *The practice of writing.* New York: St. Martin's.

Sheriden, D.R., & Dowdney, D.L. (1989). *How to write and publish articles in nursing.* New York: Springer.

Strunk, W.J., & White, E.B. (3rd ed.). (1979). *The elements of style.* New York: Macmillan.

Swanson, E., McCloskey, J., & Bodensteiner (1991). *Publishing opportunities for nurses: A comparison of 92 U.S. journals. Image–Journal of Nursing Scholarship, 23*(1), 35–38.

Tornquist, E.M. (1986). *From proposal to publication (an informal guide to writing about nursing research).* Menlo Park, CA: Addison-Wesley.

Webster's new world college dictionary (3rd ed.). (1989). Englewood Cliffs, NJ: Prentice Hall.

Zinsser, W.K. (1983). *Writing with a word processor.* New York: Harper Row.

Zinsser, W.K. (1989). *Writing to learn: How to write and think clearly about any subject at all.* New York: Harper Collins.

Zinsser, W.K. (45th rev.). (1990). *On writing well: An informal guide to writing non fiction.* New York: Harper Collins

*Highly recommended

Answers to Self-Test Questions

LESSON 1

1. FALSE. Try another journal (if appropriate) if you have a slightly different slant.

2. TRUE. When you think you have your idea defined in your mind, then do an annotated bibliography to provide some depth.

3. FALSE. The main consideration is on whom do you wish to make the greatest impact.

4. FALSE. Authors should scan the literature within the previous two years and study in depth the more recent issues.

5. FALSE. After you have established your credibility in your profession and the health care field, then go after the American consumer.

6. FALSE. Old topics can be interesting if presented with new and timely information.

7. FALSE. Term papers generally provide no new information. They generally report what has already been published.

8. TRUE. It also must be well written and presented.

9. FALSE. See the program through completion and then report it.

10. FALSE. Most papers presented verbally need some reworking in the transition from spoken word to written word.

LESSON 2

1. FALSE. The purpose of exploring library sources is to enhance your understanding of the topic even if you don't include the material in the article.

2. FALSE. General reference works provide information on subject areas, but don't depend on them for substantive content for your article.

3. TRUE. Periodical indexes and library holdings are excellent resources.

4. FALSE. You should consult with librarians whenever necessary as they are there to help you.

5. TRUE. Key words are the "key" to successful computer searches.

6. TRUE. Both computer searches and indexes and holdings can provide similar results, but a computer run-off may have greater access and will save you time if you're not in a hurry. It's a good idea to check the latest journals for up-to-date content.

7. FALSE. Compiling your working bibliography precedes your notetaking.

8. FALSE. Quoting directly is used only when (1) the person's remarks carry more weight, (2) accurate phrasing is more important, and (3) the language of the expert is more colorful, descriptive, or forceful.

9. FALSE. Authors of articles should not depend on tape recorders except in longer profile stories, oral histories, or unusual situations.

10. FALSE. Your first obligation is to the person you interview.

LESSON 3

1. TRUE. Employing the senses—sight, sound, smell, feel, and taste—will enhance the description of a person, place, or object.

2. FALSE. How you develop a narrative depends on your purpose. You may prefer to begin at the end point of a situation, back track, and then lead up to the initial starting point.

3. FALSE. More often than not, exposition assumes a supporting role through its various forms.

4. TRUE. Generally, it is presented in the imperative mood to suggest a participating audience.

5. FALSE. Comparison/contrast is often used with other expository forms, such as exemplification, analogy, or classification.

6. TRUE. First you will have to study the items to be classified and select the basis for your classification.

7. FALSE. When employing definition, you must initially identify the class or group to which the term belongs.

8. FALSE. Objectivity and your supporting evidence are the key factors.

9. TRUE. Make sure, however that a cause and effect relationship does exist.

10. FALSE. Your choice of point of view will depend upon the personal or impersonal nature of your topic and the relationship you wish to establish with your readers.

LESSON 4

1. FALSE. You may have some idea of how to proceed, but you will need a long period of sifting of data to determine how they relate before organizing into categories.

2. TRUE. Your reader is your first responsibility.

3. FALSE. Although you probably will be able to ascertain the length, the main purpose is to assemble related facts and other information to point out their similarities.

4. FALSE. The order will depend upon the nature of the subject. If inference or reason is indicated, the writer will impose logical order.

5. FALSE. Even if you have some idea of what you want to write, most of your thinking has yet to be done.

6. TRUE. It will expedite your writing because it forces you to think out your plan thoroughly beforehand.

7. TRUE. It ensures that you have firmed up your thinking and all the data are collected before beginning your article.

8. TRUE. At the outset, they define the central message of the article from which all supporting data flow.

9. FALSE. Try to consolidate your headings as much as possible. The criteria will depend on the importance of the headings and their relevancy to your subject.

10. FALSE. Your outline may be a splendid guide, but some minor changes might be indicated during the writing stage.

LESSON 5

1. FALSE. Waiting until you complete your outline will firm up your topic.

2. FALSE. Manuscripts take longer to read and may not be what the editor wants.

3. FALSE. Ethically, you should accept the assignment from only one editor.

4. TRUE. The editor may offer constructive suggestions for modifying or altering your focus.

5. FALSE. It will look more professional to type the letter.

6. FALSE. You should be familiar with the style of the three formats and how they are used.

7. TRUE. A brief proposal will give immediate visibility to your topic.

8. FALSE. Every journal carries the editor's name. Take the time to look it up.

9. TRUE. The editor may have other pressing commitments before getting to your letter.

10. FALSE. You can give a general idea, but an exact date may commit you to an unrealistic deadline.

LESSON 6

1. FALSE. Unfortunately, many leads are dull but the article still gets into print. There is no guarantee it will be read.

2. TRUE. Sometimes you have to see the entire draft before deciding on the introduction.

3. FALSE. Readers must be informed from the outset or you may lose them.

4. FALSE. Not always because it can be overworked. Use a quote when it is relevant and will draw your audience.

5. TRUE. A well presented example that is realistic will appeal to the reader.

6. TRUE. You should have a good idea of your approach even though you may wish to modify or add to your original choice.

7. FALSE. Your conclusion is your last opportunity to let the reader assess the work as a whole. A poor conclusion will detract from the article.

8. FALSE. In some cases, it is appropriate to include it toward the end of the body of the article.

9. TRUE. This is a trend in some journals and should be remedied unless the purpose of the publication changes.

10. FALSE. The writer has considerably more flexibility in non-research journals.

LESSON 7

1. TRUE. People who think clearly should be able to write clearly.

2. FALSE. A sentence that contains two or more distinctly separate thoughts lacks unity and misleads the reader.

3. FALSE. This is a common error in sentence structure of beginners.

4. FALSE. They tend to distract the reader because of choppiness and failure to build up thought.

5. TRUE. They help to build up organized thinking but do not distinguish between the importance of connected statements.

6. TRUE. They also are useful when you need to compare or contrast, or emphasize certain areas.

7. FALSE. Writers have high and low peaks but you must persevere.

8. TRUE. Some writers prefer other methods.

9. TRUE. The free flow keeps the words and thoughts coming at a fairly rapid pace without having to worry about mechanics.

10. FALSE. Unless you're a real "pro," the average number of drafts is from three to five.

LESSON 8

1. TRUE. These are the two most important elements.

2. FALSE. Although that is your expectation, you must ensure that your paper has presented new, timely, and significant information.

3. TRUE. There may be some reshuffling of headings, however, when you start revising.

4. FALSE. The body of the paper must sustain the momentum with good development.

5. TRUE. It can hurt the article.

6. FALSE. It is the quality of the content and not the quantity that counts.

7. TRUE. They build on the topic sentence.

8. FALSE. Your punctuation affects your style since it groups some words and separates others.

9. TRUE. Careless spelling will turn off an editor.

10. FALSE. Input from too many sources can confuse you.

LESSON 9

1. FALSE. It is bad form to send a manuscript to more than one journal at a time.

2. FALSE. Rejected articles are often discarded unless the author includes a stamped, self-addressed envelope.

3. TRUE. Include only citations used in the text.

4. FALSE. Some do, but the majority give extra copies of the journal tear sheets, or reprints.

5. FALSE. Blind review occurs with a little more than 50 percent of manuscripts.

6. TRUE. Copy editors deal mainly with matters of style and proofing.

7. TRUE. In the long run, it serves as a good benchmark for fostering higher quality of manuscripts.

8. TRUE. The editor's wisdom and judgment are the key factors.

9. FALSE. Only a minority have come up through the ranks.

10. FALSE. You have a perfect right to inquire after a reasonable time.

Part 2

Your Assignments: What You Need to Know

*T*he assignments in *The Writer's Notebook* represent your homework in this program and relate to each step in the writing process. They will guide you toward a publishable article if done correctly. In carrying out your assignments, you set you own deadlines as well as create your own writing lifestyle. The more you persevere, however, the sooner your article will reach fruition.

To assist you to reach your goal, the editorial staff of *Publishing for Health Dimensions (phd)* will be glad to critique your assignments and provide you with prompt and constructive feedback. *phd* aims to keep you "on track," proceeding in an orderly way. Each assignment must be completed before proceeding to the next one. If your work does not meet the expected standard, *phd* will help you until it is acceptable. However, if you choose not to use the services of *phd*, we urge you to do the assignments on your own.

Assignment 1 requires identifying the central focus of your proposed article. Because this step is so critical, *phd* is willing to advise you on your idea at a nominal charge of $10. As a bonus, you may duplicate the assignment sheet and submit two additional suggestions for articles using the same format.

To maintain continuity with your editorial expert, it is recommended that beginning authors consult on all assignments. *phd*, however, will be happy to confer with clients, particularly published authors who may wish assistance on selected assignments, such as outlining or revision. (See special fee schedule.)

In preparing assignments in *The Writer's Workbook,* you will learn the logical pattern of developing an article. Once you begin to publish, and progress from one article to the next, you will find that these steps in the writing process come more easily and naturally.

phd looks forward to working with you and helping to advance your career through writing.

Cordially,

Shirley H. Fondiller, EdD, RN

Barbara Jo Nerone, APR
Principals, *phd*

YOUR ASSIGNMENTS: WHAT YOU NEED TO KNOW

PUBLISHING FOR HEALTH DIMENSIONS 605 WEST 112 STREET • SUITE 5D • NEW YORK, NEW YORK 10025 • TELEPHONE (212) 663-4557

PLEASE RETURN THIS FORM TO THE ABOVE ADDRESS
AUTHOR INFORMATION

NAME _____

HOME ADDRESS _____

CITY _____ STATE _____ ZIP CODE _____

TELEPHONE (preferred) _____/_____ LAST EARNED DEGREE _____

POSITION TITLE _____

AGENCY _____ LOCATION _____

HAVE YOU EVER PUBLISHED? YES _____ NO _____

TITLE OF PREVIOUS PUBLICATION(S) IN LAST 2–3 YEARS. GIVE NAME, DATE, JOURNAL AND/OR BOOK TITLE, PUBLISHER, YEAR: (Use other side if needed)

CHECK THE FOLLOWING PREFERENCE:

_____ I would like to enroll in the entire program of 9 assignments.............. $69.95

_____ I would like *phd* to critique only Assignment #1 at this time.............. 10.00

_____ I will decide later if I want feedback on other assignments.

_____   _____
Date   Signature

(Kindly make out check to:
PUBLISHING FOR HEALTH DIMENSIONS)
Thank You

133

PUBLISHING FOR HEALTH DIMENSIONS-*phd*

SPECIAL FEE SCHEDULE

(Available only through *The Writer's Workbook*)

ASSIGNMENTS

#1.	Focusing on an Idea	$10
#2.	Developing an annotated bibliography	5
#3.	Developing your approach and point of view	5
#4.	Organizing your material and preparing a detailed writing outline	15
#5.	Preparing a query letter and summary of a proposed topic	10
#6.	Writing the first draft (from "catchy lead" to logical conclusion)	20
#7.		
#8.	Revising the manuscript	25
#9.	Finalizing the article for submission to a journal	10

PUBLISHING FOR HEALTH DIMENSIONS

605 WEST 112 STREET • SUITE 5D • NEW YORK, NEW YORK 10025 • TELEPHONE (212) 663-4557

NAME _____ **DATE** _____

ADDRESS _____ **CITY** _____ **STATE** _____ **ZIP** _____

TELEPHONE (Bus.) _____/_____ **(Home)** _____/_____

ASSIGNMENT 1

Please answer the questions below on this form and use extra sheets as necessary. Refer to the text for assistance.

1. *What is the central thrust of your article?*
   Identify your thesis statement by addressing the following:

   a. *Describe your topic*

   b. *Why is your point important?*

   c. *How will you present it?*

   d. *What is your point?*

   e. *Define your thesis which has evolved from your topic and questions b to d.*

2. *Who is the audience you wish to reach?*
Be specific as to health professional and type of position (i.e., staff nurses, clinical specialists, hospital administrator, physical therapy educator, and so on).

3. *What journal(s) would then be appropriate?*
Be familiar with the journal(s) and author requirements before responding.

4. *Is your article marketable?*
Address the following points:

   a. *Your proposed article has not appeared in print, particularly in recent months.*
   You have scanned the literature in the past 2 to 3 years, and more recently in depth.

   b. *Your article provides new information.*
   Identify if there is a recurring theme. If so, does your article offer a new dimension or perspective?

   c. *Your article contains significant information.*
   Indicate why you think readers will be interested in your article.

   d. *Your article is relevant.*
   Indicate why you believe your topic is timely.

YOUR ASSIGNMENTS: WHAT YOU NEED TO KNOW

e. *Your article is manageable.*
   Be certain that your expectations for completing the proposed work are realistic. You will find the time since your topic is neither too global nor complex.

5. *Do you have the expertise/qualifications to write this article?*
   The topic should be based on your experiential and/or academic background.

6. *What are your sources of information?*
   Identify if the article will be based mainly on experience, on interviews (with whom), or on types of journals, books, and other sources.

7. *How long will the manuscript be? 8 pages, 10 pages, 12 or more?* (double spaced, $8\frac{1}{2} \times 11$)
   You have checked the journal(s) of your choice for the suggested number of pages as well as author information sheet.

8. *Do you expect to use photos, charts, graphs, or other visuals?*
   Look over the journal(s) of choice for the types of visuals used. Also review author information sheet.

phd LOOKS FORWARD TO RECEIVING YOUR ASSIGNMENT. THE EDITORIAL EXPERTS WILL CAREFULLY REVIEW IT AND RETURN THE EVALUATION AND FURTHER DIRECTION WITHIN 10 TO 14 DAYS. IN THE MEANTIME, CONTINUE YOUR READING IN *THE WRITER'S WORKBOOK.*

ASSIGNMENT 2

This assignment is divided into Parts A and B. Part A includes data that you may wish to incorporate into your article. Part B is for *phd,* if you desire feedback on the assignment.

Part A—For Participants Only

1. Use 3 × 5 index cards for preparing your *Working Bibliography* as suggested in the text.

2. Use 4 × 6 index cards for *notetaking* as suggested in the text.

3. Develop an *annotated bibliography* based on items 1 and 2 above. Please follow these directions:

    a. Use white sheet typed (or word processor), 8½ × 11.

    b. Double space all copy.

    c. Copy each citation from source index card (3 × 5) in APA style. Begin with author's last name in alphabetical order.

    d. Summarize the essence of your notes from index cards (4 × 6).

    e. Annotate each citation in no less than three sentences, and no more than four or five.

4. Review the annotated bibliography. It may help you to formulate headings that will be useful for outlining later.

SEE NEXT PAGE FOR PART B

YOUR ASSIGNMENTS: WHAT YOU NEED TO KNOW

PUBLISHING
FOR HEALTH
DIMENSIONS 605 WEST 112 STREET • SUITE 5D • NEW YORK, NEW YORK 10025 • TELEPHONE (212) 663-4557

NAME _____ DATE _____

ADDRESS _____ CITY _____ STATE _____ ZIP _____

TELEPHONE (Bus.) _____/_____ (Home) _____/_____

ASSIGNMENT 2

Part B—For Participants and phd

1. Follow instructions for Part A number 3 only. Develop an *annotated bibliography*. Attach your bibliography to this sheet.

2. Describe below your *thesis statement* developed in Assignment 1.
    My thesis statement for the article is:

    _____

    _____

    _____

    _____

    _____

    _____

3. Indicate if you plan to interview authorities for your article. __ yes __ no __I don't know

4. Identify potential authorities to be interviewed:

phd LOOKS FORWARD TO RECEIVING YOUR SECOND ASSIGNMENT. THE EDITORIAL EXPERTS WILL CAREFULLY REVIEW YOUR ANNOTATED BIBLIOGRAPHY AND RETURN THE EVALUATION WITHIN 10 TO 14 DAYS. CONTINUE YOUR READING OF LESSON 3 IN *THE WRITER'S WORKBOOK.*

YOUR ASSIGNMENTS: WHAT YOU NEED TO KNOW

ASSIGNMENT 3

Please use a separate sheet of paper, typed double spaced.

1. You now should have some idea of how to develop your article. Indicate the methods you would like to use and your rationale for selecting each one. Be as specific as you can at this stage of your article.

2. Describe the dominant point of view you expect to use in your article. Explain your reasons for this selection.

3. Indicate the journal(s) of choice (for your article), and in a paragraph or two summarize the more common methods of development as well as the point of view. It is not necessary to discuss article by article.

SEE NEXT PAGE

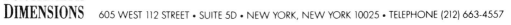

**PUBLISHING
FOR HEALTH
DIMENSIONS** 605 WEST 112 STREET • SUITE 5D • NEW YORK, NEW YORK 10025 • TELEPHONE (212) 663-4557

NAME _____ DATE _____

ADDRESS _____ CITY _____ STATE _____ ZIP _____

TELEPHONE (Bus.) _____/_____ (Home) _____/_____

ASSIGNMENT 3

Please return this form with your assignment

Describe below your *thesis statement* developed in Assignment 1:

My thesis statement for the article is:

_____

_____

_____

_____

_____

_____

_____

_____

phd LOOKS FORWARD TO RECEIVING YOUR THIRD ASSIGNMENT. THE EDITORIAL
EXPERTS WILL CAREFULLY REVIEW YOUR METHOD(S) OF DEVELOPMENT AND
POINT OF VIEW AND RETURN THE EVALUATION WITHIN 10 TO 14 DAYS. CON-
TINUE YOUR READING OF LESSON 4 IN *THE WRITER'S WORKBOOK.*

YOUR ASSIGNMENTS: WHAT YOU NEED TO KNOW

ASSIGNMENT 4

Please use a separate sheet of paper, typed double spaced.

1. Prepare a detailed writing outline of your proposed article. Develop the outline according to the introduction, body, and conclusion. Short, complex sentences are suggested.

2. Use the check list in the text to evaluate your outline.

SEE NEXT PAGE

**PUBLISHING
FOR HEALTH
DIMENSIONS** 605 WEST 112 STREET • SUITE 5D • NEW YORK, NEW YORK 10025 • TELEPHONE (212) 663-4557

NAME _____ DATE _____

ADDRESS _____ CITY _____ STATE _____ ZIP _____

TELEPHONE (Bus.) _____/_____ (Home) _____/_____

ASSIGNMENT 4

Please return this form with your assignment.

phd LOOKS FORWARD TO RECEIVING YOUR FOURTH ASSIGNMENT. THE EDITO-
RIAL EXPERTS WILL CAREFULLY REVIEW YOUR OUTLINE AND RETURN THE
EVALUATION WITHIN 10 TO 14 DAYS. CONTINUE YOUR READING OF LESSON 5 IN
THE WRITER'S WORKBOOK.

YOUR ASSIGNMENTS: WHAT YOU NEED TO KNOW

ASSIGNMENT 5

Please use a separate sheet of paper.

1. Draft what you consider an appropriate letter of query to the editor of the journal where you wish to publish your article.

2. If you plan to query more than one editor, do a draft of these letters also.

3. Prepare the letter on letterhead if you expect to use it. Be sure to use the correct format as explained in the text. Since the letter is a draft, double space it.

4. On a separate sheet (plain white paper), draft a summary of about 75 words (unless the journal or guidelines indicate otherwise) of your proposed topic. Attach this summary to the query letter or include your proposal within the letter itself.

Keep in mind that all completed letters are done in single space with double space between paragraphs.

PUBLISHING
FOR HEALTH
DIMENSIONS 605 WEST 112 STREET • SUITE 5D • NEW YORK, NEW YORK 10025 • TELEPHONE (212) 663-4557

NAME _____ DATE _____

ADDRESS _____ CITY _____ STATE _____ ZIP _____

TELEPHONE (Bus.) _____/_____ (Home) _____/_____

ASSIGNMENT 5

Please return this form with your assignment.

phd LOOKS FORWARD TO RECEIVING YOUR FIFTH ASSIGNMENT. THE EDITORIAL
EXPERTS WILL CAREFULLY REVIEW YOUR OUTLINE AND RETURN THEIR EVALU-
ATION WITHIN THE NEXT 10–14 DAYS OF RECEIVING IT. CONTINUE YOUR READ-
ING OF LESSON 6 IN *THE WRITER'S WORKBOOK.*

YOUR ASSIGNMENTS: WHAT YOU NEED TO KNOW

ASSIGNMENTS 6–7

Assignments #6–7 encompass the content in Lessons 6 and 7.

Please use separate sheets of paper.

1. Suggest two possible leads for your article and make them fairly brief. Double space on one sheet.

2. Prepare a first draft of your article following your outline. The paper should be typed triple space with the left and right margins 1½ inches each.

3. Send the above to *phd* if you wish a critique. *Please include your outline.*

PUBLISHING FOR HEALTH DIMENSIONS   605 WEST 112 STREET • SUITE 5D • NEW YORK, NEW YORK 10025 • TELEPHONE (212) 663-4557

NAME _____ DATE _____

ADDRESS _____ CITY _____ STATE _____ ZIP _____

TELEPHONE (Bus.) _____/_____ (Home) _____/_____

ASSIGNMENTS 6–7

Please return this form with your assignment.

phd LOOKS FORWARD TO RECEIVING THIS ASSIGNMENT. THE EDITORIAL EX-PERTS WILL CAREFULLY REVIEW YOUR DRAFT AND LEAD SENTENCES AND RE-TURN THE CRITIQUE WITHIN 14 DAYS OF RECEIVING IT. CONTINUE YOUR READING OF LESSON 8 IN *THE WRITER'S WORKBOOK.*

YOUR ASSIGNMENTS: WHAT YOU NEED TO KNOW

ASSIGNMENT 8

Please use a separate sheet of paper.

1. Prepare a second draft of your article, focusing on the *content* and *organization*. Follow the criteria in the text for these elements only. Be as thorough as you can.

2. If you feel comfortable about working on your style and punctuation after completing item 1 above, do so. Otherwise, wait until your next draft.

3. If you have not already submitted an outline of your paper to *phd,* do so with this second draft if you wish a critique.

**PUBLISHING
FOR HEALTH
DIMENSIONS** 605 WEST 112 STREET • SUITE 5D • NEW YORK, NEW YORK 10025 • TELEPHONE (212) 663-4557

NAME _____ **DATE** _____

ADDRESS _____ **CITY** _____ **STATE** _____ **ZIP** _____

TELEPHONE (Bus.) _____/_____ **(Home)** _____/_____

ASSIGNMENT 8

Please return this form with your assignment.

phd LOOKS FORWARD TO RECEIVING YOUR EIGHTH ASSIGNMENT. THE EDITO-RIAL EXPERTS WILL CAREFULLY REVIEW YOUR SECOND DRAFT AND RETURN THE CRITIQUE WITHIN 14 DAYS OF RECEIVING IT. CONTINUE YOUR READING OF LESSON 9 IN *THE WRITER'S WORKBOOK*.

YOUR ASSIGNMENTS: WHAT YOU NEED TO KNOW

ASSIGNMENT 9

Please use a separate sheet of paper.

PART A. YOUR THIRD DRAFT

1. Prepare a third draft of your article, incorporating the suggestions from *phd* on your second draft.

2. Refer to the text in LESSON 8 and test again for content and organization, refining your previous drafts.

3. Next, TEST FOR STYLE AND CLARITY OF EXPRESSION, addressing the questions about words and sentences.

4. TEST FOR MECHANICS

IF YOU ARE NOT READY FOR PART B, DO PART A ONLY

PART B. YOUR FOURTH DRAFT (POSSIBLY YOUR FINAL DRAFT)

1. Prepare the manuscript as if you are now ready to send it to the editor of your target journal. Follow the guidelines for authors of the journal.

2. Do a draft of the cover letter to the editor to be included with the manuscript.

3. Indicate if photos or visuals are to be included. (Do not send to *phd*).

**PUBLISHING
FOR HEALTH
DIMENSIONS** 605 WEST 112 STREET • SUITE 5D • NEW YORK, NEW YORK 10025 • TELEPHONE (212) 663-4557

NAME _____ **DATE** _____

ADDRESS _____ **CITY** _____ **STATE** _____ **ZIP** _____

TELEPHONE (Bus.) _____/_____ **(Home)** _____/_____

ASSIGNMENT 9

Please check:

Yes _____ No _____ Enclosed is a 3rd draft (Part A) of my article.

Yes _____ No _____ Enclosed is a 4th draft (Part B) of my article.

Yes _____ No _____ I have obtained outside feedback on my manuscript.

IDENTIFY THE PERSON BELOW:

Name _____

Title _____

Credentials _____

Please return this form with your assignment.

phd LOOKS FORWARD TO RECEIVING YOUR NINTH ASSIGNMENT. THE EDITORIAL EXPERTS WILL CAREFULLY REVIEW YOUR THIRD & FOURTH DRAFTS AND RETURN THEIR CRITIQUE WITHIN THE NEXT 14 DAYS OF RECEIVING IT. CONTINUE YOUR READING OF LESSON 10 IN *THE WRITER'S WORKBOOK.*

Part 3

Do's and Don'ts
of Modern Usage

A. HOW TO ELIMINATE COMMON ABUSES

1. *Use Modifiers Properly.* Modifiers must be placed so that they modify the right words or phrases.

a. *Misplaced Modifier*

Poor: *He decided when he had finished the assignment to quit.*

In this sentence, what does *when he had finished the assignment* mean? To modify *decided* or *to quit?*

Both sentences 1 and 2 below read clearly depending on the intent.

Improved: 1. *When he had finished the assignment, he decided to quit.*

or

2. *He decided to quit when he had finished the assignment.*

b. *Dangling Modifier*

Poor: *Checking the medication cabinet, the demerol bottle was missing.*

Improved: *Checking the medication cabinet, the nurse couldn't find the demerol bottle.*

2. *Avoid Ambiguous Statements*

Poor: *Mary's supervisor says that she will be working a longer shift today.*

Who will work the longer shift? Mary or the supervisor? The correct intent is stated below.

Improved: *According to her supervisor, Mary will work the longer shift today.*

3. *Accentuate Active Verbs*

Active verbs give vitality to writing, whereas the passive voice tends to dull prose.

Poor: *Since the methodology was faulty, the study's results were inconclusive.*

Improved: *The study showed inconclusive results because of faulty methodology.*

4. *Watch That Jargon!*

Jargon is obscure and often pretentious language, characteristic of a special group or activity.

Poor: *He prepped the patient for surgery.*

Improved: *He prepared the patient for surgery.*

5. *Reduce Repetition of Words*

Words repeated at the beginning of consecutive sentences should be avoided unless the repetition is for emphasis.

Poor: *Ms. Stewart showed the patient how to use the propenal inhaler. The inhaler was a new treatment for asthma. Asthma is an increasing health problem among Americans.*

Improved: *Ms. Stewart showed the patient how to use the propenal inhaler, which is a new treatment for asthma, an increasing health problem among Americans.*

6. *Avoid Converting Verbs Into Nouns*

Do not change verbs to nouns ending in *tion, tive, ance, ment.*

Poor: *He proposed the course for the advancement of his profession.*

Improved: *He proposed the course to advance his profession.*

7. *Keep Your Verb Close to the Subject*

Poor: *Pam and Jo, driving to the conference during a torrential storm, agonized over the treacherous curves.*

Improved: *Driving to the conference during a torrential storm, Pam and Jo agonized over the treacherous curves.*

8. *Use Consistent Tense*

   Poor: *Dr. Bennett discussed the test results, which show that learning took place.*

   Improved: *Dr. Bennett discussed the test results, which showed that learning took place.*

9. *De-emphasize Sexist Language*

   Whenever possible, use the plural form to avoid the generic use of masculine or feminine pronouns. If inappropriate, employ the gender representing the majority of the group or category described. Avoid use of he/she or his/her unless the publication you write for requests this usage.

   Poor: *A health professional cannot use knowledge that he doesn't have.*

   Improved: *Health professionals cannot use knowledge that they don't have.*

10. *Avoid Cliches*

    Poor: *The program featured a think tank of experts on health policy.*

    Improved: *The program featured experts on health care policy.*

B. HOW TO SIMPLIFY YOUR LANGUAGE

   In the two columns below, the first one contains the preferred words. Although similar in meaning, the phrases or words in the opposite column appear more frequently and should be avoided as much as possible.

Preferred	*Avoid*
if	in the event that
because	due to the fact that
frequently	it is often the case that
believe	be of the opinion
although	in spite of the fact that
before	in advance of
was	had occasion to be
consider	take into consideration
indicate	in indicative of
now	at the present time
to	in order to
help	facilitate
pattern	paradigm
when	during the time that

C. HOW TO ELIMINATE REDUNDANCY

In the commonly used examples below, one (or two) of the words should be removed.

temporary reprieve	spell out *in detail*	*exact* same
absolutely essential	*basic* fundamentals	refer *back* to
true fact	*completely* unanimous	eliminate *completely*
advanced planning	*each and* every	

D. HOW TO AVOID OVERUSE OF THE VERB "TO BE"

When sentences contain weak-linking verbs, such as *is, are, have, was,* and other forms of the verb "to be," they generate lazy prose. In a few steps, the following exercise shows you how to eliminate this problem with all *5 verbs* removed.

Original Version

This small monograph *is* an excellent summary of current concepts of physical assessment. It *is* profusely illustrated with beautiful pictures and clean diagrams. The test *is* relatively simple and *is* obviously written for the non-expert, for there *are* few references cited.

Step 1. In the first sentence, substitute an active verb so that the sentence reads as follows: *This small monograph summarizes excellently the current concepts of physical assessment.*

Step 2. Eliminate *is* in the second sentence, and combine the first and second sentences to read: *Profusely illustrated with beautiful pictures and clean diagrams, this small monograph summarizes excellently the current concepts of physical assessment.*

Step 3. Sentence 3 becomes sentence 2. Eliminate the three uses of the verb "to be,"—*is, is, are*—and substitute the active verb *cites* for *cited.* The sentence now reads: *Obviously written for the non-expert, the relatively simple text cites few references.*

Corrected Version

Profusely illustrated with beautiful pictures and clear diagrams, this small monograph summarizes excellently the current concepts of physical assessment. Obviously written for the non-expert, the relatively simple text cites few references.

Isn't it easy when you know how? Practice the principles involved in the above process and you will improve your style and clarity of expression.

Common Proofreader's Marks

Mark	Meaning	Mark	Meaning
ℐ	Delete	◡	Close up; delete space
ℐ (with close up)	Delete and close up (use only when deleting letters *within* a word)	⊙	Insert period
¶	Begin new paragraph	⌄ (comma)	Insert comma
⊏	Move left	⌄ (apostrophe)	Insert apostrophe (or single quotation mark)
stet	Let it stand	⌄⌄	Insert quotation marks
tr	Transpose	;/	Insert semicolon
(sp)	Spell out	:/	Insert colon
lc	Set in lowercase (uncapitalized)	(set) ?	Insert question mark
cap	Set in CAPITAL letters	|=|	Insert hyphen
bf	Set in **boldface** type	⌐N⌐	Insert en dash
ital	Set in *italic* type	⌐M⌐	Insert em dash
#	Insert space	(|)	Insert parentheses

List of Nursing Journals

The Writer's Workbook expresses its appreciation to *Image-Journal of Nursing Scholarship* (Volume 23, Number 1) for granting permission to reproduce the listing of nursing journals below. Published in the Spring 1991 issue, this comprehensive but succinct compendium of journal information was included in an article, "Publishing Opportunities for Nurses: A Comparison of 92 U.S. Journals," authored by Elizabeth A. Swanson, Joanne C. McCloskey, and Anne Bodensteiner.

Collected in 1990, the data show the scope of the journal market, with publications continuing to rise as nursing specialization increases. In 1977, there were 22 nursing journals! The present figure of 92 in the listing represents 80 percent to 90 percent of the actual number. Any exclusions may be due to the fact that some editors did not respond to the survey, a publication may be discontinued, or new journals have appeared since reporting the results.

Although journal requirements may alter from time to time, the specific data listed under the various categories remain fairly accurate. Publications, however, should be checked in the library for correct addresses, names and titles of editors, and other pertinent information. The library also has many health care journals that prospective writers should explore.

Name of Journal	Circulation Paid 1	Comp 2	Issues 3	Pages Year 4	Copies Ms. 5	Form++ of Ms. 6	Query* Letter 7	Free Repr. 8	Staff Write (%) 9	Solicited (%) 10	Research (%) 11
Administration											
Jnl of Nsg Administration	12000	400	11	12-15	3	a	o	12	0	25	15
Jnl of Nsg Quality Assurance	4159	94	4	20	3	a	p	0	0	20	10
Nsg Economics	6200		6	12-15	3	b	p	3		40	20
Nsg Management	120000	5000	12	10	2	c	p		10	0	10
Series on Nsg Administration			1	20	12-15	b	n		0	100	10
Advanced Clinical Practice											
Clinical Nurse Specialist	3006	700	4	10-15	5	b	o		0	5	20
Nse Prac: Am. Jnl. of Primary Health Care	8839	3700	12	15	4	b	p	2	2	10	30
The Diabetes Educator	5800	50	6	12	3	d	n		10	15	75
Education											
Jnl of Continuing Education in Nsg	4200		6	15	5	b	o	5	0	0	50
Jnl of Nsg Education	5000	150	9	15	4	b	n	5	0	0	80
Jnl of Nsg Staff Development	3443	108	6	12-16	3	b	o		0	0	10
Nurse Educator	3600	200	6	14	3	d	o		0	10	10
Nsg and Health Care	15000	500	10		4	b	o	1	15	25	30
General Practice											
Advancing Clinical Care			6	6-10	4	b	o,p	3	5	15	5
American Jnl of Nsg			12	12	2	a	p	5			
Emphasis: Nursing	0	3500	2	18	3		o	2	30	50	30
Jnl of Christian Nsg	12488	718	4	10	1		o		20	68	2
Jnl of National Black Nurses' Assoc.	2850	30	2	12-15	4	b	p	1	2		75
Jnl of Practical Nsg	9435	1200	4	8-10	1	a	p	5	10	90	
Nsg 90	506777	6704	12	10-15	3		p		0	10	0
Nsg Clinics of North America			4	20	1	e	n	100	0	0	0
Nsg Diagnosis			4	15-20	4	b	n		0	10	80
RN	255232	28414	12	5-10	2		p		1	30	1
Professional Development											
Computers in Nsg	5000		6	18	3	b	o	1	0		50
Image: Jnl of Nsg Scholarship	78750+		4	14	4	b	o		0	0	70
Imprint	18000+		5	8	2	b	o	5	5	50	0
Jnl of Professional Nsg	2000+	100	6	15-20	4	b	n	1	5	10	30
Nsg Connections	1700	100	4	14-15	3	b	o		0	5	20
Nsg Outlook	13000+	325	6	12-16	3	a	o	100	1	20	25
Scholarly Inquiry for Nsg Practice	500	45	3	20	4	b	p	1	5	5	60
Technology for Nsg	250	100	12				n		100	0	20
Research											
Advances in Nsg Science	2907	133	4	15-30	3	f		0	0	0	
Annual Review of Nsg Research			1	30	5	b	o		0	100	
Applied Nsg Research			4	8-12	5	b	o	0	0	0	100
Nsg Research	12000	150	6	14-16	3		p	0	0	0	80
Research in Nsg and Health	1653	55	6	10-15	4	b	o	50	0	0	100
Western Jnl of Nsg Research			6	15	4	b	o	2	0	1	90
Specialty Practice											
Community											
AAOHN Jnl	13500+		12	8-14	5	b	n	5	0	30	25
Caring Magazine	6000+		12	10-12	2	a	o		5	25	5
Family and Community Health	1803	86	4	15-18	3	f	o		0	60	30
Home Health Care Nurse	5500	3000	6	12	4	b	o		0	40	5
Public Health Nsg			4	10-30	3	b	o		0	0	75
School Nurse	18000+		4	10-12	1	f	o	6	0	0	10
Critical Care											
Cardiovascular Nsg	26100+		6	10-15	3	e	o	o	10	10	60
Critical Care Nsg Quarterly	4429	64	4	15-18	3	f	o	2	5	90	25
Critical Care Nurse	39305	1437	12	20-25	4	f	o	2	0	15	15
Dimensions of Critical Care Nsg	5000		6	12-20	3	f	p	3	0	20	10
Focus on Critical Care	65751+	740	6	14	4	d	p		0	5	5
Heart & Lung: Jnl of Critical Care	69900+	780	6	10-12	3	d	o	25	0	5	70
Jnl of Cardiovascular Nsg	2271	4	4	10-30	3	f			0	90	15
Jnl of Emergency Nsg	23237	543	6	7-10	5	f	o		5	95	20

LIST OF NURSING JOURNALS

Name of Journal	Circulation Paid 1	Circulation Comp 2	Issues 3	Pages Year 4	Copies Ms. 5	Form++ of Ms. 6	Query* Letter 7	Free Repr. 8	Staff Write (%) 9	Solicited (%) 10	Research (%) 11
Gerontology											
Am Jnl of Alzheimers Care &Related Disorders and Res.	2000	1000	6	12-15	3			2	0	50	60
Geriatric Nsg: Am Jnl of Care for the Aging	31000	2000	6	10-12	3		p	0	1	20	20
Jnl of Gerontological Nsg	11500	100	12	8-10	4	f	o	5	0	5	40
Holistic Nursing											
Holistic Nsg Practice	2369	102	4	15-18	3	f	o	2	0	90	20
Jnl of Holistic Nsg	2050+		1	18-20	3	b	n		10		50
Maternal/Child											
Birth	4800		4	8-10	3	d	n		0	0	70
Issues in Comprehensive Pediatric Nsg	707	15	4	15-20	2	b	o	0	5	10	100
Jnl of Nurse-Midwifery	4200+	300	6	20-30	2	e	o	1	5	10	50
Jnl of Pediatric Health Care	4500+	540	6	15	4	b	o	5	0	50	20
Jnl of Pediatric Nsg: Nsg Care of Children and Families			6		3	b	o	50	0	0	50
Jnl of Perinatal and Neonatal Nsg	3688	62	4	15-18	3	f	o	2	40	50	10
Maternal-Child Nsg Jnl	1325	50	4	25-35	3	b	o		5	5	75
Midwifery Today	1200	100	4	1-8	1		n	1	5	5	10
Neonatal Network: The Jnl of Neonatal Nsg	14350+	150	8	10-20	2	f	o		0	0	15
Pediatric Nsg	12000		6	12-15	4	b	o	2	15	15	40
Mental Health											
Archives of Psychiatric Nsg			6	16-18	3	b	o	25	1	3	40
Issues in Mental Health Nsg	926	20	4	10-20	3	b	o	1	3	20	67
Jnl of Child and Adolescent Psychiatric and Mental Health Nsg	1000	100	4	12-16	4	b	o		0	25	75
Jnl of Psychosocial Nsg	13500+	100	12	8-10	4	b	o	5	0	5	15
Nephrology											
American Nephrology Nurses Association Jnl	12000+	7000	6	15	6	b	p	0	0	40	40
Jnl of Urological Nsg	1800+		4		3	b	p	5	10	90	25
Urologic Nsg	2050+	30	4	4-12	3		o	2	1	89	8
Oncology											
Dimensions in Oncology Nsg	1200+		4	7-10	3	f	p		20	70	10
Oncology Nsg Forum	18240+	432	6	12-14	4	a	o		0	20	40
Seminars in Oncology Nsg	2300	30	4	15	2	a	p	50		100	1
Operating Room											
AANA Jnl	24953+	41	6	12-20	3	a	n		0	28	39
AORN Jnl	44000+	500	12	20	3	c	p		10	18	10
Jnl of Post Anesthesia Nsg	7301+	100	6	15-20	5		p	50	35	30	30
Today's OR Nurse	8500	100	12	12	4	f	o	5	0	25	0
Rehabilitation											
Rehabilitation Nsg	7300	350	6	4-12	4	b	o	1	0	0	50
Spinal Cord Injury Nsg	1480+	737	4	10-15	4	b	o		5	0	20
Other											
AIDS Patient Care	10000		6	10	1	e	o		50	25	10
Gastroenterology Nsg	4048+	10	4	10-15	2	d	p	1	40	10	4
Jnl of Intravenous Nsg	8000+		6	6-8	5	e	o	1	0	100	33
Jnl of Neuroscience Nsg	4900	20	6	20	5	e	o		0	10	30
Jnl of Opthalmic Nsg and Technology	4500	100	6	14	4	f	o	5	0	10	40
Jnl of Transcultural Nsg	380+	40	2	20	4	b		1	2	7	87
Laser Nsg	3000	1000	4	8	2	d	o	5	0	100	5
Orthopaedic Nsg	10800+		6	20	5	b	o	3	0	65	10
Ostomy Wound Management	13000	5500	6	12	4	e	o	5		100	25
Plastic Surgical Nsg			4	10-12	4	b	o	2	5	70	5
Society of Otorhinolaryngology & Head-Neck Nurses` Jnl	850	25	4	15	2		o		0	10	5

+   Beneift of Membership in Organization

++   Format required
     a=   Chicago Manual of Style
     b=   American Psychological Association
     c=   Turabian
     d=   Index Medicus
     e=   Journal's Own
     f=   other

*   Query Letter
     n=   not wanted
     0=   optional
     p=   preffered

THE WRITER'S WORKBOOK

Name of Journal	Unsol. Recvd. (N) 1	Unsol. Publ. (N) 2	Mss. Reject (N) 3	Acceptance Rate (%) 4	Refereed 5	Review** Proc. 6	Time Period Accepted 7	Time Period Published 8
Administration								
Jnl of Nsg Administration	223	42	181	19	y	3	2 mo	8 mo
Jnl of Nsg Quality Assurance	50	40	10	80	y	3	6-8 wk	6-9 mo
Nsg Economics	61	34	31	56	y	3	4 mo	4-6 mo
Nsg Management	1000	110	850	11		4	6-8 wk	v
Series on Nsg Administration	0				n	3	6 wk	9 mo
Advanced Clinical Practice								
Clinical Nurse Specialist	61	27	18	44	y	2	3 mo	3 mo-1 yr
Nse Prac: Am. Jnl. of Primary Health Care	120	48	72	40	y	3	2 mo	1 yr
The Diabetes Educator	48	30	14	63	y	3	6-8 wk	6 mo
Education								
Jnl of Continuing Education in Nsg	75	25	35	33	y	4	4 mo	18-24 mo
Jnl of Nsg Education	309	79	230	26	y	3	4 mo	8 mo
Jnl of Nsg Staff Development	72	14	14	19	y	3	3-4 mo	1 yr
Nurse Educator	194	40	150	21	y	3	6 wk	10 mo
Nsg and Health Care	126	28		22	y	3	2 mo	2-3 mo
General Practice								
Advancing Clinical Care	250	200	50	80	y	3	6 wk	2-3 mo
American Jnl of Nsg					y	4		
Emphasis: Nursing	18	3	40	17	y	3	4 wk	5 mo
Jnl of Christian Nsg	67	8	59	12	y	1	3-4 mo	1-2 yrs
Jnl of National Black Nurses' Assoc.	34		12		y	3	6 mo	1 yr
Jnl of Practical Nsg					y	1	up to 1 yr	up to 1 yr
Nsg 90	700	160	550	23	y	3	1-3 mo	6-12 mo
Nsg Clinics of North America	10	0	10					
Nsg Diagnosis	14	10	1	71	y	3	4 mo	3 mo
RN	424	81	321	19	y	4	2 mo	6-8 mo
Professional Development								
Computers in Nsg	200	24	120	12	y	4	6 mo	1yr
Image: Jnl of Nsg Scholarship	258	50	183	19	y	3	5-6 mo	6 mo
Imprint					n	2	1 mo	3 mo
Jnl of Professional Nsg	131	36	70	27	y	3	3.5 mo	5 mo
Nsg Connections	80	20	60	25	y	3	3-4 mo	4-10 mo
Nsg Outlook	150	33	86	22	y	3	2-3 mo	1-3 yr
Scholarly Inquiry for Nsg Practice	36	7	17	19	y	3	2 mo	6 mo
Technology for Nsg	0							
Research								
Advances in Nsg Science	200	26	174	13	y	3	8-10 wk	4 mo
Annual Review of Nsg Research							NA	24-36 mo
Applied Nsg Research	25	12	13	48	y	3	3-6 mo	6-12 mo
Nsg Research	430	65	365	15	y	3	2 mo	7 mo
Research in Nsg and Health	192	42	132	22	y	3	<=3 mo	6-9 mo
Western Jnl of Nsg Research	167	34	53	20	y	3	6 mo	1 yr
Specialty Practice								
Community								
AAOHN Jnl	65	40	9	62	y	3	2.8 mo	3.3 mo
Caring Magazine	150	100	30	67	n	3	2 mo	3-6 mo
Family and Community Health	30	12	18	40	y	3	1-3 mo	6-12 mo
Home Health Care Nurse	49	34	15	69	y	3	6 mo	3-6 mo
Public Health Nsg	150	31	64	21	y	3	2-4 mo	6-9 mo
School Nurse	26	13	5	50	y	3	6 mo	9-12 mo
Critical Care								
Cardiovascular Nsg	15	5	2	33	y	3	6-8 wk	
Critical Care Nsg Quarterly	17	6	8	35	y	3	6 wk	2 mo
Critical Care Nurse	300	100	75	33	y	3	5-6 wk	9-12 mo
Dimensions of Critical Care Nsg	102	31	61	30	y	3	7 wk	8-10 mo
Focus on Critical Care	95	19	29	20	y	3	3 mo	1 yr
Heart & Lung: Jnl of Critical Care	284	94	120	33	y	3	6-8 wk	6-8 mo
Jnl of Cardiovascular Nsg	20	5	25	25	y	3	2 mo	6 mo
Jnl of Emergency Nsg	70	40	15	57	y	3	6 wk	3 mo

LIST OF NURSING JOURNALS

Name of Journal	Unsol. Recvd. (N) 1	Unsol. Publ. (N) 2	Mss. Reject (N) 3	Acceptance Rate (%) 4	Refereed 5	Review** Proc. 6	Time Period Accepted 7	Time Period Published 8
Gerontology								
Am Jnl of Alzheimers Care & Related Disorders and Res.	20	36	7	180	y	3	3 wk-1 yr	3 wk-1 yr
Geriatric Nsg: Am Jnl of Care for the Aging	80	10	40	13	y	3	3-4 mo	1 yr
Jnl of Gerontological Nsg	250	60	120	24	y	3	5 mo	4 mo
Holistic Nursing								
Holistic Nsg Practice	30	4	12	13	y	3	3 mo	6 mo
Jnl of Holistic Nsg	17	7	1	41	y	3	3-4 mo	3-4 mo
Maternal/Child								
Birth					y	2	v	v
Issues in Comprehensive Pediatric Nsg	35	30	5	86	y	3	4-6 mo	4-6 mo
Jnl of Nurse-Midwifery	82	54	28	66	y	4	2-3 mo	4-6 mo
Jnl of Pediatric Health Care	90	48	85	53	y	3	2 mo	6-9 mo
Jnl of Pediatric Nsg: Nsg Care of Children and Families	117				y	3	6-12 wk	9-15 mo
Jnl of Perinatal and Neonatal Nsg	5				y	3	2-6 wk	6 mo
Maternal-Child Nsg Jnl	25	1	4	4	y	3	1 yr	3-6 mo
Midwifery Today	130	100	10	77	n	1	4-6 wk	3-6 mo
Neonatal Network:The Jnl of Neonatal Nsg	60	36	24	60	y	3	2-4 mo	1 yr
Pediatric Nsg	100	30	25	30	y	3	2 mo	10 mo
Mental Health								
Archives of Psychiatric Nsg	109	54	54	50	y	3	3 mo	5 mo
Issues in Mental Health Nsg	46	28	18	61	y	3	4 mo	6 mo
Jnl of Child and Adolescent Psychiatric and Mental Health Nsg.	26	14	2	54	y	3	1-3 mo	6 mo
Jnl of Psychosocial Nsg	250	60	120	24	y	3	4 mo	3 mo
Nephrology								
American Nephrology Nurses Association Jnl	30	6		20	y	3	2-3 mo	6-8 mo
Jnl of Urological Nsg	0	0	15		y	2	1 mo	pending on cont
Urologic Nsg	5	1	1	20	y	3	1-2 mo	3 mo-1yr
Oncology								
Dimensions in Oncology Nsg	5	5	7	100	y	3	6 wk	6 mo
Oncology Nsg Forum	200		40		y	3	3 mo	3-6 mo
Seminars in Oncology Nsg	2	2	2	100	y	2		
Operating Room								
AANA Jnl	60	22	10	37	y	3	1-5 mo	3 mo-1 yr
AORN Jnl	50	20		40	y	3	6-8 wk	6-9 mo
Jnl of Post Anesthesia Nsg	84	60	2	71	y	3	2-3 mo	6-12 mo
Today's OR Nurse	100	40	20	40	y	3	3 mo	3 mo
Specialty Practice								
Rehabilitation								
Rehabilitation Nsg	63	31	11	49	y		1-2 mo	6-12 mo
Spinal Cord Injury Nsg	12	8	4	67	y	3	3 mo	3-6 mo
Other								
AIDS Patient Care	40	30	10	75	n	1	1 mo	3-6 mo
Gastroenterology Nsg	29	25	4	86	y	3	4-6 mo	8-12 mo
Jnl of Intravenous Nsg					y	3	3 mo	1-3 mo
Jnl of Neuroscience Nsg	90	47	4	52	y	3	3 mo	3 mo
Jnl of Opthalmic Nsg and Technology	40	20	10	50	y	3	2 mo	2 mo
Jnl of Transcultural Nsg	5	2	1	40	y	3	2 mo	<=1 yr
Laser Nsg	5	5	0	100	y	2	3 mo	6 mo
Orthopaedic Nsg	35	12	13	34	y	3	10-12 wk	6 mo
Ostomy Wound Management	11	7	4	64	y	3	3 mo	3 mo
Plastic Surgical Nsg	7	6	0	86	y	3	2 mo	3-4 mo
Society of Otorhinolarynogology & Head-Neck Nurses' Jnl	18	12	6	67	y	3	3 mo	4-6 mo

** Review Procedure
1= Editor receives, reviews, seeks consultation from content experts if necessary, but otherwise singularly makes the decision for or against publication
2= Editor receives manuscript, reviews, and sends to associate editor responsible for content area. Associate editor reviews manusrcipts, recommends acceptance or rejection, and reaches final decision in collaboration with editor and/or other associate editors
3= Editor receives manuscripts, reviews, and distributes them to experts selected from an established group of reviewers. Decision on the manuscript is based on reviews and mediated by editor
4= Other (please explain)

—